Childbirth
with Insight

Carmen:
Thanks for coming
to the Chicago
Workshop.
Elizabeth Noble

Childbirth with Insight

Elizabeth Noble

Photographs
by Harriette Hartigan

Boston
HOUGHTON MIFFLIN COMPANY 1983

Appendixes 1, 2, 3, and 4 are based on: Roberto Caldeyro-Barcia, "The influence of maternal bearing-down efforts during second stage on fetal well-being," in *Kaleidoscope of Childbearing: Preparation, Birth, and Nurturing*, edited by Penny Simkin and Carla Reinke. Seattle: the pennypress, 1978. Reproduced with permission from the pennypress.

Appendix 5 is based on material from *Obstetrics Illustrated*, 3rd ed., edited by Matthew M. Garrey, A.D.T. Govon, C.H. Hodge, and R. Callander. London: Churchill, 1980.

Appendix 6 was prepared by Doris Haire, President, American Foundation for Maternal and Child Health; Consultant, International Childbirth Education Association, Inc. It is reprinted by permission of the author.

Appendix 7 is reprinted with permission of the pennypress, 1100 23rd Ave. East, Seattle, WA 98112.

Paul Reps's poetry is reprinted with his permission.

Library of Congress Cataloging in Publication Data

Noble, Elizabeth, date
  Childbirth with insight.

  Bibliography: p.
  Includes index.
    1. Natural childbirth.   2. Childbirth—Psychological aspects.   3. Childbirth—Study and teaching.   I. Title.
RG661.N63   1983   618.4'5   82-21326
ISBN 0-395-32518-8
ISBN 0-395-33962-6 (pbk.)

Printed in the United States of America

V 10 9 8 7 6 5 4 3 2 1

To Doris and John Haire

Acknowledgments

I am grateful to the following people for their criticism of and contributions to the manuscript: Suzanne Arms, Doris Haire, D.M.S., Judith Lasater, Ph.D., R.P.T., Eva Reich, M.D., Leo Sorger, M.D., F.A.C.O.G., Frans Veldman, and Diony Young, B.A.

My editor, Anita McClellan, deserves special mention for her thought and effort, which went well beyond the bounds of duty.

My appreciation and thanks to my husband, Geoff, and my colleagues at the Maternal and Child Health Center for their support and assistance.

Foreword

Childbirth with Insight is a pioneering book that is likely to change the direction of childbirth preparation and management. Elizabeth Noble blends together the latest understanding of the normal physiology of labor with an individualized approach to help the mother and her partner respond spontaneously to the biological mechanisms of labor. *Childbirth with Insight* brings my research and that of others to the general public in a clear, readable manner and in a context that should generate a better understanding of the normal process of birth.

I first met Elizabeth Noble at an International Childbirth Education Association conference in 1977. At that time, she questioned the wisdom of encouraging mothers to use strong, prolonged bearing-down efforts, combined with breath-holding, during the second stage (expulsive phase) of labor. She expressed her concern that instructing the mother to bear down long and hard was the more likely cause of fetal hypoxia and acidosis seen in the second stage than the length of time involved in that stage of labor. Investigations indicate that the conduct of second stage in this manner can be dangerous for the fetus.

Elizabeth Noble examines the very foundations of conventional childbirth techniques. She explores the effects of controlled breathing during the various phases of labor from both a psychological and a physiological perspective. In doing so, she points out that many human biological processes do not lend themselves to prolonged control without adverse effects and that a flexible approach based on body awareness is essential to a safe and satisfying childbirth.

Technological advancement in medicine continues to provide valuable tools for the obstetrician. However, we must not fail to observe and appreciate the intricate checks and balances of nature. There should be no interference with the normal process of labor without good reason. Recent studies have indicated that the mother's self-regulation of her position, breathing, and bearing-down in labor lead to improved outcome, biochemically as well as emotionally.

Childbirth education plays an important role in the continual improvement of maternity care. Elizabeth Noble's contribution has been to emphasize the normal physiology of childbearing, and in this book, she adds a philosophical dimension. The unique feature of this book is that it is not oriented to a specific method. Thus, it has broad appeal to and application for every expectant couple. Both professionals in the field and expectant couples will find the new ideas in *Childbirth with Insight* enlightening and encouraging.

Roberto Caldeyro-Barcia, M.D.

Immediate Past President, International Federation of Gynecologists and Obstetricians

Former Director, Latin American Center for Perinatology and Human Development, World Health Organization

Professor and Director, Department of Perinatology, Faculty of Medicine, University of the Republic, Montevideo, Uruguay

Contents

Introduction

A Return to Fundamentals

THE LITERATURE on childbearing is already formidable. Books on birth are getting thicker all the time, carrying titles that promise encyclopedic coverage. Many authors value gathering new obstetrical information, however patchy or superficial, more than integrating or conveying an understanding of what we already know about the mind and body during childbearing. Therefore, fundamental aspects of the childbirth process are buried under a mass of data and professional controversy.

Childbirth calls into question our very existence, requiring an expectant couple to confront not only new life but death, pain, fear, and most of all, change. In *Childbirth with Insight* I will attempt to help couples in their exploration of these issues. In addressing the physiological and psychological aspects of childbirth preparation, this book will involve your basic assumptions about life, health, the mind, and the body. Looking at birth philosophically as well will provide a better understanding of the influences of our cultural attitudes on the miracle of pregnancy and birth. Our exploration will concern insights that are not just intellectual but emotional. We will be looking at ways to acknowledge deep feelings and to deal with the fear and anxiety attendant on birthing.

The medical and general literature lacks clear and simple descriptions of what happens physiologically in a wom-

. . . The experience of pain, of sickness and of death [is] an integral part of [man's] life. The ability to cope with this trio autonomously is fundamental to his health.
IVAN ILLICH

Knowledge becomes understanding when it is coupled with feeling.
ALEXANDER LOWEN

an's body during childbirth. However, plenty has been written about techniques and procedures. Birthing women need to be encouraged simply to integrate their minds with their bodies in order to cooperate with the natural forces acting within themselves during pregnancy and birth. Instead, they are generally trained and exhorted to struggle against their bodies' involuntary reflexes and intense feelings in the name of a particular method of childbirth preparation learned in six or eight weeks.

The emphasis of *Childbirth with Insight* is on normal birth, which is possible for the overwhelming majority of women. Unfortunately, most women's potential for normal, healthy childbearing has been obscured by medical and media preoccupation with the abnormal aspects of labor and technological interference (often referred to as "progress") in the natural birth process. The medicalization of birth is relatively recent; Jimmy Carter was the first U.S. president to be born in a hospital. Yet the American College of Obstetricians and Gynecologists has called homebirth the "earliest form of child abuse."

The preference for unnatural childbirth practices, which seems to be spreading across the world, despite countermovements to tune into the natural process, has led birth, in many places, to be a major psychological disaster zone, in which almost everything is done the exact opposite way from how it would happen if allowed to.
R. D. LAING

Studies have shown that the hospital is not safer than the home for low-risk births. Moreover, hospital birth environments have been traditionally repressive. In the United States, particularly, surgical specialists attend women during childbirth. Indeed, the very substance of American obstetrical education, as opposed to the schooling of midwives, emphasizes deviations from what medicine considers the norm. Physicians in residence may never witness a normal labor or delivery. No wonder caesarean rates are skyrocketing. Medical intervention in birth is widespread; midwifery and homebirth are often restricted or even outlawed.

Because parents are transients in the maternity care system, there is little cumulative birth experience over successive generations of mothers. Women giving birth don't make the same mistakes as their mothers or grandmothers — they make new ones. Even women whose birth knowledge is provided by female relatives and family experience, rather than books and prenatal classes, are not prepared for the "no risk, high-tech" medical handling of birth today. If this tide of intervention is not turned back soon, it will become increasingly difficult for a pregnant woman to trust her intuition in order to give birth according to her feelings and insights, rather than by the prescriptions of a specific birth method.

The renaissance of midwifery is an encouraging sign. More and more women are coming to realize that, unless they have found an exceptional physician, they have a much greater chance of natural birth with a midwife. Some midwives, of course, are heavily influenced by hospital practices and view pregnant women as patients. Ideally, one should seek a midwife who has a deep trust in the process of birth and the skills to keep labor normal, unraveling any problems before they become complications requiring medical intervention.

Most incredible of all, is the ready acceptance by a woman of those whose guidance and care is sought in childbirth.
GRANTLY DICK-READ

Birth in a Broader Context

Childbirth educators, usually the spokespersons for mothers and babies, criticize the specific obstetric practices but usually do not question the larger framework that fosters the medicalization of birth. Childbirth instructors are aware of political and economic questions surrounding hospital birth, such as high fees, medical prestige, male power, and the falling birth rate. Like their medical counterparts, most childbirth educators are trapped in a philosophical void in regard to wider questions about human existence and the interaction between a person's conscious and unconscious processes. Moreover, childbirth education has contributed artificial guidelines and techniques to explain and structure the birth process for expectant parents. Preparation for childbirth, like medical training, focuses on the tools of the trade, rather than developing a couple's understanding not only of birth but of life itself. Childbirth education, based on the classroom model, schools expectant parents in what professionals think they need to know, instead of encouraging a couple's holistic learning and self-exploration. Holding on to old methods means that more and more labors will be made to fit the medical opinion that birth requires intervention to be successful. Restructuring childbirth education should help to reduce the ever-increasing rate of caesareans.

Birth does not happen in isolation. It is part of a continuum not only of the childbearing year but of a woman's lifetime. Pregnancy triggers an expanded state of consciousness that readies a woman for personal growth and lifestyle changes. This heightened awareness nurtures a woman's bond with her baby and prepares her for motherhood. Pregnancy and birth provide a couple with the perfect opportunity for self-discovery; a special chance to develop greater appreciation of the interaction of mind, spirit, and body and the pleasures of living. A woman naturally lives more in the present during the maternity cycle, looking inward, becoming more in touch with deep feelings, and communicating with her unborn child. The actual birth is a journey into the unknown, just as life is a journey into the unknown — an adventure to look forward to, if a woman can flow with it spontaneously.

The most that we in the helping professions can hope to do is to present expectant couples with a few guiding principles, while respecting the physiology of labor and the individuality of each birth. It is important for childbirth instructors to review any teachings that may be unphysiological, counterproductive, or psychologically harmful to childbearing women. Any modification of a woman's birth behavior, however well intended, should be regarded as potential intervention. The positions and procedures that are most routinely imposed on the birth process are also those that most need to be questioned. Professionals and consumers demand data and documentation about the effects of drugs or electronic fetal heart monitoring on mother and baby. The same insistence also applies to documentation about the effects of labor techniques that alter a woman's physiology and emotional response, such as controlled breathing patterns. (In a recent letter to *Whole Life Times*, a mother listed the inventory of well-known labor interventions and added that women are also "made to breathe like idiots.") My concern here is not whether one set of rules and regulations for labor is better than

To be fulfilled is to be filled full, and that means a full belly whether of good food or good feeling.
ALEXANDER LOWEN

another but that there can be *no* appropriate method, or any outside control, of such an individual experience as birth.

Avoiding "Trendy" Techniques

Criticism of the status quo may unintentionally lead to new techniques and dogma. Dr. Frederick Leboyer made a powerful plea for more sensitive handling of the newborn in his book and film *Birth Without Violence*. While his message was universally acclaimed, among professionals there was a lot of fussing about trivial details, such as how to sterilize the water for a newborn's bath, what exact temperature it should be, and so on. Technicalities became more important than emotions.

Our vision of the universe is lost in the overwhelming complexity of details.
ALAN WATTS

In *Essential Exercises for the Childbearing Year*, first published in 1976, I explain the role of key muscles during each phase of the maternity cycle. Logically, this included labor and delivery. These explanations raised questions about the conventional handling of birth, specifically, control of the breath. Childbirth educators and birth attendants became intrigued with my explanation that the breath should be released while the abdominal muscles shorten during effort. Such breathing is nothing more than efficient respiratory and body mechanics, be it during childbirth, sports, or any form of physical exertion. Women, if free to be spontaneous, generally breathe out with groaning sounds during the expulsive phase of birth, or even at other times during labor.

A physiological reflex that has existed as long as humankind cannot be claimed by anyone as a new technique developed for a particular method of childbirth instruction. Nonetheless, soon after the publication of *Essential Exercises for the Childbearing Year*, all sorts of acclaim (and, of course, the occasional condemnation) was heard for the "new pushing technique," "Noble's method of exhale pushing," "forced exhalation," "trumpet-blowing," or "gentle pushing." This was similar to considering a description of what happens to the heart and lungs in running a newly developed, breakthrough method for joggers!

Because I was asked to present numerous workshops and lectures on alternative pushing, I delved further into the physiology and psychology of breath-holding during exertion. The more I learned the more I knew that the conventional management of second-stage labor is, as R. D. Laing would say, "an effort of 180° in the opposite direction, without insight." (Dr. Roberto Caldeyro-Barcia has since conducted the research that scientifically puts to rest the question of bearing-down with a closed glottis. See page 64.)

Moving from Control to Freedom

The key is understanding. To ask how to do this, what is the technique or method, what are the steps and rules, is to miss the point entirely.
ALAN WATTS

Maternity staff and birth partners find it difficult to encourage a laboring woman to let go of her breath and body only in the second stage of labor, if the whole of first-stage labor has been an exercise in mental control, outer-directed effort, and coached breathing. Inevitably, my work led me to evaluate the practice of controlled breathing at any time in labor and ultimately to question the idea of control itself — during birth and during life.

It is time to examine the whole forest, instead of inspecting individual trees. The experience of birth is much larger than the sum of its parts. The more we reduce those parts for detailed analysis and programming the more we lose sight of birth in all its dimensions. *Childbirth with Insight* explores philosophical assumptions underlying control, change, fear, the nature of personal freedom, and the relation between mind, body, and the emotions. Such scrutiny is fundamental in order that providers and consumers of childbirth preparation and labor support go beyond token or piecemeal adjustments to their labor programs. A

It is not just a matter of seeing things differently but of seeing different things.
MARILYN FERGUSON

new, holistic perspective on childbirth is necessary and will make a complete reversal of childbirth education inevitable. This does not mean more knowledge but a "new knowing," as Marilyn Ferguson phrases it in *The Aquarian Conspiracy.* Childbirth educators and maternity staff can benefit from exciting new transformations occurring in all levels of society, through a whole range of informal networks. Rather than defending past practices because they were trained to use them, childbirth professionals, like expectant couples, need to learn for themselves how to let go of restrictive beliefs and attitudes. If change and innovation can be seen as a challenge rather than a threat, then childbirth with freedom and insight will be possible.

By considering more physiological alternatives to current birth methods and by exploring psychological dilemmas of conventional childbirth preparation, I am not advocating a new educational method. It would be to my everlasting regret to have inadvertently fostered yet more teaching techniques to add to the array that complicates childbirth preparation today. There is nothing new about the way women give birth, only about the way that those around them control the birth environment and the experience.

Childbirth with Insight is a philosophical inquiry and a guide to a variety of resources and approaches for living in the here and now. It is not a manual on giving birth. Writing about "how to" achieve a goal rather than about understanding the process of living and being oneself would be a contradiction of my purpose. My intent is to find ways to unite and simplify childbirth preparation so that couples can share their childbearing experiences with more insight and laboring women can act in accordance with their individual needs.

A vision can be realized in many ways . . . a goal in only one.
MARILYN FERGUSON

Childbearing integrates a woman's mind and body in the most intense way and brings on an existential crisis. However, this crisis is instructive rather than destructive. It forces a woman to rethink the meaning of her life, and to deal with the imminent, inevitable changes of lifestyle and family roles. During pregnancy and birth, women have the opportunity to decide for themselves whether the theories of science, philosophy, and medicine part company with their own knowledge and insights. Women may experience birth with heightened awareness and pleasure or they may bring fear or unresolved conflicts to their labor and get stuck in the process. Women's fear of the intensity of labor, in a society that values rational thought and control, has led to widespread belief that bodily sensations can be masterfully blocked by the power of the mind.

A couple's ability to discover and seek their own style of birth is limited when prescribed behavior restricts spontaneity and creates anxiety about performing to an observer's set of standards. Human response is more creative than ideas of certainty and predictability permit. It is not easy for any of us to transcend years of habit and social conditioning, especially when most childbirth education courses reinforce the unfortunate assumption that the mind is separate from and superior to the body. More and more people are looking into holistic health and personal growth movements that recognize the integration of mind, body, and feelings. On the other hand, childbirth preparation classes still emphasize lectures that are easier to structure than experiential sessions where couples explore their bodies and emotions. As such, prenatal classes are an extension of traditional education where mental skills are developed and refined at the expense of physical and emotional awareness. Family history, especially attitudes and beliefs, influences pregnancy and birth outcome and must also be considered in holistic childbirth preparation.

The human being is not a thing but a process, not an object but life.
ALAN WATTS

Various therapies, such as Haptonomy, hypnosis, Rebirthing, Primal Therapy and Natal Therapy, as well as psychiatrists such as R. D. Laing and Stanislav Grof, have stressed the crucial significance of the prenatal existence as well as the birth experience in shaping an individual's entire life. Ironically, such insights were made by those who do not work in obstetrics and are rarely known or appreciated by health care professionals who do work with pregnant women. New approaches typically come from outside a discipline, because experts are usually limited by their own training and close familiarity with their fields. My own growth, personal and professional, has meant letting go of much of my formal education in order to effect a synthesis of ideas gleaned from diverse fields.

Childbirth educators can help foster a couple's creativity and self-confidence to give birth in their own special way.

Expectant parents need to understand the normal physiology of labor, to increase awareness of their bodies and feelings, and to develop self-reliance. They also have a tremendous need for support to enable them to desire natural childbirth and to feel comfortable about taking responsibility for birth back from medical experts, hospital attendants, and obstetric technology. By giving birth normally, without interference, a couple greatly increases their self-esteem and sense of individual power and independence. Such a foundation is invaluable for happy and healthy childrearing. Parents who are in touch with themselves and their bodies are able to raise their children with trust, respect, and close physical contact, thus nurturing individuals who will bring joy and peace to our troubled and violent world.

Self-actualizing people have a wonderful capacity to appreciate again and again, freshly and naively, the basic goods of life with awe, pleasure, wonder and even ecstasy, however stale these experiences may be for other people.
ABRAHAM MASLOW

Resources

Ferguson, Marilyn. *The Aquarian Conspiracy: Personal and Social Transformation in the 1980s.* Los Angeles: Tarcher, 1980. An inspirational book dealing with the power of individuals and informal networks for change.

Leboyer, Frederick. *Birth Without Violence.* New York: Knopf, 1975. The classic that pioneered the humanization of birth and gentle handling of the newborn.

————. *Inner Beauty, Inner Light: Yoga for Pregnant Women.* New York: Knopf, 1977. A poetic book emphasizing the natural and spiritual aspects of pregnancy and birth.

Noble, Elizabeth. *Essential Exercises for the Childbearing Year.* Second ed., Revised. Boston: Houghton Mifflin, 1982. Describes the role of key muscles (the abdominals and pelvic floor) through pregnancy, birth, and postpartum. Emphasizes women's understanding of their bodies; details preventive and restorative exercises, including after caesarean birth.

Two bookstores specializing in mail-order books on pregnancy, birth, and parenthood are:

Birth and Life Bookstore, P.O. Box 70625, Seattle, WA 98107.

ICEA Bookcenter, P.O. Box 20048, Minneapolis, MN 55420.

Mail-order books, tapes, and records on holistic health and personal growth can be obtained from:

Association for Research and Enlightenment, Inc., P.O. Box 595, Virginia Beach, VA 23451.

Childbirth
with Insight

CHAPTER 1

Childbearing from a Philosophical Perspective

QUESTIONS ABOUT birth inevitably raise questions about life. Fundamental beliefs and attitudes are usually unconscious, although they affect the whole range of our behavior. Childbirth affords an opportunity for a couple to examine assumptions about themselves, the world, life and death. If we review ideas, both personal and social, that orient us to our daily existence, we can better understand their implications and limitations. Such introspection and questioning of belief systems tends to be characteristic of Eastern cultures and is a growing influence on the human potential movement and holistic therapies of contemporary Western society. The integration of these approaches expands the dimensions of obstetrics and enriches preparation for birth.

At the basis of the whole modern view of the world lies the illusion that the so-called laws of nature are the explanations of natural phenomena.
LUDWIG
WITTGENSTEIN

The Universe in Constant Flux

Our understanding of our bodies, our minds, of nature and reality, is constantly being challenged by scientists and philosophers. The more we learn about the universe, the more it is clear that we live in a world where all phenomena are interrelated and nothing can be isolated or regarded as absolute.

Progress in natural science has forced a reconsideration

The world flows along; our system of reference breaks it up.
ALAN WATTS

of the most basic scientific and philosophic concepts. Time is not linear and "solid" matter is actually a mass of moving particles. Mechanical rules from the old physics, such as Newton's laws, still serve us on an everyday level but are too limited to deal with galaxies and electrons. As Fritjof Capra points out in *The Tao of Physics*, quantum, relativity, and systems theories have forced modern researchers to see that the world is just as Eastern mystics have surmised for centuries. This new perspective is holistic, appreciating the interconnectedness and uncertainty of the whole cosmic system. *Life force* and *universal energy* are not just esoteric phrases but help describe the physical universe. Such scientific insights have been the subject of popular books and television programs. Carl Sagan's *Cosmos* and Jacob Bronowski's *The Ascent of Man* have brought some of the most advanced concepts into millions of living rooms. Nonetheless, most people continue to view the universe, like the human body, as a machine with a collection of measurable and predictable parts. This mechanical view is reductionistic. Looking at smaller parts of the whole yields an incomplete picture. It is not possible to separate the observer from what is being observed; so controlled studies and "objective" experiments can only provide a partial answer to a limited hypothesis.

Because knowledge is gained in pieces, we forget that reality is not like that.
ALAN WATTS

Researchers are discovering that human consciousness is even more complex and rich in potential than they ever imagined. Each half of the brain contributes different aspects of consciousness, although the left side, which controls intellect and goal-oriented performance, is typically more developed in people who live in industrialized societies. The left brain analyzes and recognizes; it is the seat of mathematical and verbal skills. The right brain, which Marilyn Ferguson terms the "heart-brain," functions in dreaming, intuition, holistic awareness, creative expression, and pain mediation. These faculties tend to be underused by people in our technological era. Pregnancy and birth tune women in to the functions of the right brain, which has a multitude of connections with the limbic system or "visceral brain." This older and more primitive part of the nervous system influences biological rhythms, sexual behavior, motivation, and emotions such as fear and rage. The limbic system is also involved in altered states of consciousness and is the seat of primal pain and pre-verbal experience.

The Mechanical Model of Medicine

Recent scientific discoveries and holistic insights appear to have had little impact on medicine. Technological innova-tion in health care remains a priority and runs parallel with an increasingly automated way of life. Patients' bodies are viewed like the workings of a clock, with parts that can be fixed or even replaced. Research studies continue to be based on a mechanical view of both the universe and the human body. Most doctors search for single causes of dis-eases, or perhaps one or two risk factors, instead of seek-ing out an individual's pattern of health and illness over time. Medical remedies, too frequently restricted to drugs and surgery, address the symptoms rather than the whole person. The nature and functioning of the body parts be-come the focus for medical investigation, while physicians lose sight of other dimensions of disease, such as beliefs and emotions.*

Human values get lost in a mechanistic world. Medical students are brought up to believe that every problem has a solution, that every service has a provider. With that kind of arrogance, it is no wonder that we are short of honesty, affection and real usefulness.
KERR L. WHITE

Obstetric training and childbirth education continue to operate in a limited, linear framework. The sequence and nature of events in the childbearing year are considered to be orderly and manageable with medical expertise. A pregnant woman is not often treated as a whole person, with body, mind, and feelings. Instead she may be la-belled "the breech coming in at three P.M." (referring to the position of her baby when the lower part presents first for birth instead of the head), or "an arrested labor in room four" (referring to a woman's slowed or stopped contrac-tions). Instead of expressing interest in why or how these situations have evolved, professionals try to decide which

If we depend too much on machines, we become machines ourselves.
FREDERICK LEBOYER

---

* The placebo effect (patients experiencing relief or cure from a dummy treatment) is well accepted in medicine, yet the broader implications for improving health through changing belief systems has been little appre-ciated.

intervention will engineer the woman's machinery "back on course."

Along with the traditional view of a "pill for every ill" is the medical profession's commitment to medical triumph over the forces of nature. Conventional medicine may be losing the war against cancer (considered by many to be a holistic disease*), but it won't be long before babies will be grown in artificial incubators instead of the uterus. At that point the most natural and transcendental human experience will be reduced to a laboratory technique. Nevertheless, ethics and the origins of consciousness will continue to elude medical control.

Unfortunately, a great many people share the medical establishment's mechanistic view that control of nature is good and that progress is only a matter of *more* — more pills, more techniques, more information. This contrasts with the new holistic attitude in science that more and more technology will not solve the problems that plague our world today. As Dr. Robert Mendelsohn writes in *Confessions of a Medical Heretic*, the password of physicians is "above all, do something." This medical positivism ignores the interaction of mind and body in the quest for short-term clinical results. Understanding the deeper questions is rarely a priority for either party, as patients themselves often press doctors for a quick fix.

Patients may not realize that when they reject the technological route of modern medicine, they need to develop faith in a holistic approach. This requires self-awareness, self-reliance, perhaps great courage. In *Anatomy of an Illness*, Norman Cousins describes how, with the assistance of vitamin C, he laughed himself free of a severe joint disease. By suspending rational belief in a mechanistic treatment, he substituted a holistic approach, akin to mysticism, which was successful. In *Mind and Matter*, Dr.

The more time, toil and sacrifice spent by a population in producing medicine as a commodity, the larger will be the by-product, namely, the fallacy that society has a supply of health locked away which can be mined and marketed.
IVAN ILLICH

* In *Getting Well Again*, Dr. Carl Simonton and his team profile the typical "cancer personality" and describe the psychological strategies that have been very successful at their Cancer Counseling and Research Center in Fort Worth, Texas. In June 1982, the National Cancer Institute released a major scientific report, *Diet, Nutrition and Cancer*, associating long-term eating patterns with the development of the most common cancers.

Lewis Mehl presents many case histories in which he worked with clients holistically to help resolve such illnesses as diabetes and asthma. More conventional ways of dealing with uncertainties in medical treatment, including birth and death, can be found in *Medical Choices, Medical Chances,* written by a group of doctors as a guide for consensual decision-making.

People overlook the fact that in addition to their conscious thoughts, their brains are coordinating countless simultaneous bodily functions. These include respiration, digestion, excretion, circulation, and the most miraculous of all, the growth of a baby. This self-regulation of the body is unappreciated until the "machinery" fails. Only when the medical repair shops can't take care of headaches, allergies, or other ailments are people forced to consider the way they use and abuse themselves. Then interest is kindled in physical functioning and emotional well-being. Some decide to "jog the body" or to put stiff joints through yoga postures. But bodies are what people *are*, not what people have. Any physical transformation, as holistic practitioners well know, has to occur in both body and mind. Likewise, emotional release can dramatically change posture, facial expressions, and other body language.

The medical model of disease considers people victims attacked by viruses or infections at which the treatment is directed. Because we objectify our bodies, we "make" love, "have" orgasms, "catch" a cold, or "get" diabetes. Diseases are always expressed as nouns — things that happen to us. Yet all of us participate, consciously and unconsciously, in our health and sickness. Likewise, labor is the product of a process. That process is a woman and her surroundings. Labor is not something that happens to a woman, it is the result of a woman and her child working together for birth.

Although childbearing is a normal process, it is treated by many professionals as a disease. In fact, the application of high-tech intervention in birth and the fragmented mechanistic treatment of laboring women is increasing with fervor, especially in industrialized countries' major medical centers. (Many modern practices involving women and children — such as feeding infants prepared formula rather than breast milk — are being exported to Third World countries with serious medical and economic consequences.) Despite the growth of midwifery, home-birth, and feminist self-help health care movements, elaborate technology and complex procedures appear to make medical experts even more knowledgeable and valuable. Thus, physicians become more desirable to the uninformed consumer of maternity services than midwives, and nonchildbearers continue to oversee the childbearers. As a result of all the new machinery developed for use in obstetrics, hospital labor and delivery areas increasingly resemble intensive-care units. Ultrasound, fetal monitoring, scalp blood sampling, and the increasing caesarean rate make it easier for hospitals to recruit residents in obstetrics and gynecology* — now a high-powered surgical specialty. Although midwives have less technological and academic training, they observe the whole of labor, offering time, patience, and an appreciation of the family unit.

Women today rely on the props of drugs, machines and other people instead of relying on themselves and their bodies to do the work of labor.
DIONY YOUNG

The mechanistic model of medicine affects maternity care in many ways. For example, women are told that there is a prescribed length of each stage of every labor and many physicians insist on a fixed weight gain for all their pregnant clients. Statistical average is used to determine birth norms (the Friedman labor curve is one such tool) while the whole range of normal birth limits is overlooked. Such maps and measurements obscure reality and the natural variation in human beings and may cause great disservice to parents and newborns.

The map is not the territory.
ALAN WATTS

Holistic medicine, on the other hand, raises questions that many would prefer to leave unasked. It demands flexibility, interest in environmental influences, family interaction (not just disease history), and a commitment to the uniqueness of each individual. Ripples of change are start-

---

* The American Medical Association has predicted that there will be a surplus of more than 10,000 obstetricians by 1990. In the meantime, the AMA has called upon family practitioners to attend 25 percent of births to keep obstetrics under physician control and out of the hands of midwives.

ing to spread from fringe health movements into the mainstream of health care consumers. Educational training is now offered by organizations specializing in holistic approaches, and holistic medical groups are growing in popularity. Many people are becoming tired of the mechanistic approaches of conventional medicine and want to close the gap between mind and body. This is not to suggest that technology be abandoned but that it be united with a humanistic approach. It is like putting on a new pair of glasses to see the whole picture.

The Body-Mind Problem

Our mechanistic culture classifies, compares, and sees the universe in terms of parts, rather than as a constantly changing continuum. We live in a polarized world; earth versus cosmos, human versus nature, men versus women, and mind versus body. Indeed, a pervasive gap between body and mind is at the root of medicine's mechanical approach. Psychiatrists concern themselves only with the mind, whereas a whole gamut of physical specialists look after the body. Experts on the workings of bodily parts tend to deny the role of feelings, and psychotherapists often discount the language of the body.

We think of ourselves as minds that have or live in bodies. The mind becomes the rider, in control, while the body is the horse — to be trained and used.
JOEL KRAMER

Psychotherapists and social workers constitute a high proportion of clients seeking back and neck treatment, for what they view as a mechanical breakdown in the body, divorced from feelings and lifestyle. As yoga instructor and physical therapist Judith Lasater expressed it, "it's as if they chose a profession where they could study objectively what they cannot experience subjectively." In fact, professionals at either end of the body-mind spectrum set great value on detachment and objectivity. By objectifying a client, they do not see the whole person. In turn, clients present either their bodies or their psyches, but not their complete selves.

In my own practice, I treat a lot of spinal problems. Mobilization of the joints is usually successful in just a few sessions. However, patients often return in about two years with a relapse, sometimes in the same area, at other times a little lower or higher in the spine. Many surgeons would remove the offending disk. Chiropractors typically repeat mechanical body techniques for months and even years. The more any therapist becomes committed to a holistic approach, the more he or she is forced to admit that underlying emotional factors are showing up as tension, stiffness, or a painful "weak spot."

When direct clinical treatment fails, less mechanical therapies that involve the mind as well as the body, such as Bioenergetics, Radix, Primal Therapy, hypnosis, and visualization, often succeed. Massage can also be cathartic. Reflexology focuses on the feet or hands for systemic effects. In psychoperistaltic massage (developed in England by Gerda Boyesen), the masseur or masseuse listens to intestinal sounds with an electronic stethoscope while working on the client's body. Rolfing* is very deep massage to attempt to bring about a realignment of the body. These massage experiences can be time-consuming and are resisted by left-brain people who want a reductionistic diagnosis and an instant cure. Dr. Alexander Lowen, an early pioneer in Bioenergetics, points out that the most common tension syndromes — depression, low back pain, and myopia — are virtually accepted as normal just because they are so universal.

The Haptonomic approach, developed by Frans Veldman in the Netherlands, is one of the least threatening and most pleasurable of the personal growth therapies. Based on scientifically proven powers of touch, the client learns to develop emotional security through the release of involuntary muscle tension. As the client is able to extend the limits of his or her body, he or she can interact with greater freedom and awareness. Haptonomy allows one to easily and quickly experience the sense of what it is to "be" there as a whole person.

Many of us discover in adult life that we feel less than whole, that the "feeling" part of us has been buried under

---

* Some Rolfers massage too hard. Dr. Eva Reich points out that pain is not healed by more pain. More is gained by melting the armor than by trying to break it.

all kinds of pressure and preoccupations. This forced repression begins in childhood and has been lucidly described by Richard Farson in *Birthrights*. Social development causes us to experience ourselves as separate entities, a mind apart from a body, left-brain functions at the expense of those of the right brain, and learned behavior camouflaging feelings. A sense of self is not only a mental experience. We experience thoughts and emotions on a bodily level as well, such as the goose flesh of fear or blushing with embarrassment. Parts of the self are expressed in the body as chronic muscular tensions, affecting posture and behavior. For every individual pattern of muscular contraction, there is a corresponding repressed emotional state without which such tension would not exist. Contraction of muscles, voluntarily controlled in childhood and puberty initially, creates a feeling of physical power and control over various sensations and emotions. "Armoring" of the body thus blocks primal pain. As adults we perpetuate the cycle in our power play with children because we cannot stand to be reminded of our own loss of self. Bioenergetics and Radix are based on Wilhelm Reich's observation that an individual's character is expressed in his or her body armor.

Human beings begin their lives as butterflies and end up in cocoons.
MARILYN FERGUSON

Bodily events in a person's lifetime also affect psychological growth, just as rejection, deprivation, and other emotional trauma are reflected in tension laid down in the body. We have all learned to present certain behavioral patterns, which are reinforced by family and teachers, and to keep the rest of ourselves hidden. Our greatest socialization for bodily control concerns the intimate functions of the excretory and genital organs. The pelvic area, particularly with regard to sexuality, is most likely to resist mental dominance and thus requires the most effort for suppression. Throughout a person's development, sadness and crying are held back. The abdominal-pelvic cavity is one place where these emotions become bottled up and it is also the area where energy accumulates for sexual release. For many people, sex is a limited release of genital tension rather than a positive, whole-self expression of sexual feeling. Little girls in particular are taught to repress

The function of the orgasm becomes the yardstick of psychophysical functioning because the function of biological energy is expressed in it.
WILHELM REICH

rather than to respond to any sensations "down there," as Nancy Friday points out in her unsettling book *My Mother, My Self.*

There is no place to get in touch with the feelings during pregnancy. In childbirth classes, they say education will take care of the fear but they don't deal with it. "Anne," in The World of the Unborn *by* LENI SCHWARTZ

Sexual repression can be doubly damaging for women who choose to bear children, as it is in the pelvic area that pregnancy and birth are experienced. Birth, like sex, involves powerful and spontaneous expression. Feelings and emotions are therefore very important for a woman to consider during her childbearing year. We create the meaning of events in our life and select the ways we react to them, albeit often unconsciously. There are no wrong feelings; there are just feelings. Feelings bias our attention and can affect brain chemistry. They can explain, and even resolve, some of the technical diagnoses during pregnancy, birth, and postpartum. Some midwives know this well. If contractions slow down or stop, they will speak of a woman "closing down," rather than using the medical term *uterine inertia.* More than one mother, comparing birth experiences with a midwife and an obstetrician, has recalled the midwife's encouraging "bring your baby into the world" in contrast with the doctor's commands to *"push, push."* Intuitive birth attendants understand that a woman's own birth can affect how she gives birth.* Many primal emotions surface during labor — or get stuck — and in both cases the process of birth is affected. Breast-feeding difficulties usually arise from the mother-child relationship rather than from problems with the mother's milk that would require a switch to prepared infant formula.

Holding in feelings to maintain self-composure is an unhealthy way to try to be brave. It takes more courage to be who we are, particularly when surrounded by disapproval from medical experts who think they know more about us than we know about ourselves. By understanding how her defense mechanisms work, a mother can more easily explore how she internalizes emotions such as fear and disappointment. One example is reaction to stress. Our

* In *Realms of the Human Unconscious* psychiatrist Stanislav Grof observes how mothers reliving their own births under LSD therapy could not tell if they were being born or giving birth themselves.

ability to cope with stress largely depends on decisions made in childhood, when, as a reaction to our parents, we pledged to ourselves "never" or "always" to behave in a certain fashion. Some people under stress continue to put others first, some explode, some withdraw, and others cover one emotion with another. It is essential for an expectant mother to let her feelings surface and to trust in the wisdom of her body, if she is to become the unique person that her potential promises. By becoming free herself, she will have the confidence to allow her child freedom and autonomy. Instead of protecting her child like a possession, she will protect her child's *rights* to be a self-regulating human being from birth.

Free, self-regulated behaviour fills people with enthusiasm, but at the same time, it terrifies them.
WILHELM REICH

The Paradox of Control

We live in a society bent on unilateral control, whether it be of the Russians, the gypsy moths, or the second stage of labor. Most childbirth educators present structured techniques to guide expectant parents toward a particular form of behavior during labor. The appeal of any given method of birth is that the prescriptions and formulas appear to make the birth experience predictable and manageable. This control not only suits hospitals, physicians, and educators but many pregnant women as well. The promise of control resonates with a woman's fear and anxiety about birth and falsely suggests that her mind and body function as separate entities.

In a typical controlled labor, the mother works against her body in the name of "prepared childbirth," although this educational birth intervention is taught with the best of intentions. Rehearsed and resolute, the laboring woman stares at a focal point and paces her breathing through different patterns of pants and blows in an attempt to keep her pain out of her mind. Her knuckles turn white as she grips the side rails of the bed. As contractions become more intense, she deliberately accelerates her breathing over the peak, determined to stay on top of the pain and of the situation. The labor gets tougher and the mother becomes more fatigued, yet she valiantly struggles to pace her breathing and focus her vision to dissociate herself from her body. While she is fragmenting her consciousness and energy with this busy-work, she also worries about how well she is performing the techniques and coping with her ordeal. Looking around for approval from the maternity staff, she asks, "Am I doing it right?" "Should I change breathing to another level now?"

Anxiety appears when deep in ourselves we know that we have no other choice, no alternative way of acting.
MOSHE FELDENKRAIS

Her partner, briefly trained as her coach, feels very inadequate by this time, especially if his recommendations conflict with those of the staff or if she is showing signs of "losing control" that he cannot remedy.

If the mother is confined to bed with typical hospital interventions such as an intravenous drip or electronic fetal heart monitor, her labor will be made longer (without the assistance of gravity and movement) and more painful (if she is lying on her back). Denied nourishment, she is probably hungry and thirsty as well. Low blood sugar, overbreathing, and narcotics lead to the dizziness, nausea, and trembling that are considered characteristic of the "transition" phase of labor.

After the mother's cervix is fully dilated, the second stage of labor is typically heralded by birth attendants' chorus of "push, push, push!" The mother is reminded to hold her elbows away from her side and to fix her ribs and diaphragm by holding her breath. At the same time she is expected to relax the rest of her body selectively. This is impossible: Her arms are holding up her legs as she is flexing her upper body against the force of gravity. As her eyes bulge and her face turns purple, her pelvic floor muscles protectively tighten against increasing intra-abdominal pressure. The baby's head is forced uphill through a tense perineum; an episiotomy is cut to enlarge the mother's vaginal opening. The undue exertion required for a laboring woman to perform the techniques that "being in control" demands can become very tiring and contribute to delay or difficulties with her labor. Thus, many women are too exhausted to carry on in second stage. Also, the birth may not be moving fast enough for the obstetrician ("failure to progress") and anesthesia, in-

A sense of futility of life, tiredness and a wish to give it all up is the result of overtaxing the conscious control with tasks that the reflexive and subconscious nervous activity is better fitted to perform.
MOSHE FELDENKRAIS

struments, or even caesarean delivery will be employed to complete the birth.

Most hospital births today, and most childbirth education films, depict at least some of the forementioned interventions, both medical and educational. Prepared childbirth films, with few exceptions, are instructive rather than enlightening. They confirm a particular teaching method by advocating roles and techniques. Such films obscure the fundamental holistic experience of birth. Couples are not aware that the power of giving birth involves individual surrender to its uncontrollable nature. It is understandable that expectant parents become anxious about their abilities to maintain the kind of control that is expected of them, given that no such control of natural forces is possible — or desirable.

The actual experience of contractions, like other intense bodily sensations, is extremely difficult to describe. A woman forgets the contraction as soon as it passes. The physical experience overwhelms her mind and memory. The more completely an expectant mother can experience labor as a unit of mind and body, the more easily she can flow with the process of birth. As one mother said afterward, "I didn't know I could have just gone with the pain. I thought I had to escape from it, to fight it." The more a woman tries to be in control, the more she fears the inevitable loss of control, which leads to feelings of guilt and failure.

When laboring women are not centered on themselves and working harmoniously with their bodies, they become spectators rather than participants in their own birth experiences. Feeling anxious or self-conscious inhibits spontaneity. The most joyful experiences of life happen of their own accord. Loving, laughing, absorption in something interesting, all involve living in the here and now. As the late philosopher Alan Watts pointed out, the preoccupation with sex in our society is an attempt to make up for the lack of spontaneity in all other dimensions of modern existence.

As long as the mind believes it is possible to escape from what it is at this moment, there can be no freedom.
ALAN WATTS

The important thing is what we are doing, and not what we have to do.
B. K. S. IYENGAR

Adapting to Change

Growth means change; old ways die and new ones emerge. This process cannot be willed — things leave us when we are ready to release them, including the fear of change and the desire for control.

Mostly people think of change in their lives as an end in itself. If we can adjust to one major shift, we should be set for good. But change is an ongoing process, a fact of human existence, a continual death and rebirth. Everyone's life has another hurdle to jump, another fork in its road.

The more we become ourselves, the more we change.
CARL ROGERS

Increased awareness of their bodies helps people to feel more complete. Solutions to the unexpected are then more creative and appropriate to individual needs. Self-reliance derives from confidence in the self-regulation of our bodies and the humble appreciation of the place humans hold in the universe. We feel extremely helpless if sickness or injury forces a radical change in our lives. But opportunity lies within every crisis and adaptation yields greater flexibility as we meet the unpredictable. The bamboo bends in the storm; the oak will break. Seeing ourselves as part of an ever-changing and dynamic universe helps to remind us that as creatures we were meant to adapt, and adaptation is crucial to human growth and survival.

A belated discovery, one that causes considerable anguish, is that no one can persuade another to change. Each of us guards a gate of change that can only be unlocked from the inside. We cannot open the gate of another, either by argument or by emotional appeal.
MARILYN FERGUSON

Human beings are capable of an enormous range of cultural and physical change. An experience that causes premature aging in one individual, like a divorce, may cause amazing rejuvenation in another. One person diagnosed with cancer will slowly let himself die, while another with the same type of cancer will take steps to cure or regress the disease and live on with renewed vigor.

Fear of the Unknown

Every expectant couple worries about how to handle the stress and pain of labor. Anxiety before any new and intense event is normal and healthy. Such emotions serve to mobilize the pregnant woman to take care of herself, to become well-informed, and to make the necessary preparation for her birth.

It is essential for a mother to make a strong commitment to natural childbirth and to seek support for this decision from friends, family, childbirth educators, midwives, and physicians.* An expectant mother needs to find a supportive environment that permits her to respond as she wishes during birth. Likewise, she should remove herself from people who undermine her confidence, even if this involves a family member or requires changing her physician or midwife in late pregnancy.

Conventional childbirth education emphasizes a mother's control and practice of her planned performance. Yet a woman needs to make peace with all her fears and to shape realistic expectations for her birth and motherhood experience. Learning about "certainty" doesn't help her deal with uncertainty. To counterbalance the pressure for mental control, every pregnant woman needs to get in touch with her physical self, to deepen her consciousness of her body's sensory experience and her accompanying emotions. The more threatened a woman may feel by the alien physical changes during her childbearing year, the more she needs to come to terms with her body. When comfortable with her physical self, and with her full consciousness, a woman in labor will move naturally in ways that will help her to flow with contractions and to release any mental resistance to them. Only then can she be guided by the individual tugs and pulls of her own labor rather than by prescriptions learned in prenatal class and rehearsed before the actual event.

Pregnant women often worry about how they will behave — or "misbehave" — in labor, especially if they have an ideal model in their mind, introduced or reinforced by childbirth preparation films and classes. Con-

The other side of every fear is freedom.
MARILYN FERGUSON

Control over persons and things is rejected in favor of a deep and sympathetic insight into the self and others.
CARL ROGERS

---

* Pessimists may comment that one should not aspire to natural childbirth in case complications develop. This is like saying one shouldn't bond with the baby in case it dies, or one shouldn't fall in love in case one gets hurt. Such timidity and antilife sentiments lead to self-fulfilling prophecies and deny the human potential to respond to the unexpected.

cern about animalistic behavior, antisocial noises, soiling
the sheets or attendants, is very deep. Crying or other
expressions of release or suffering are seen as signs of
weakness and are shameful because the self is not being
presented in its everyday role. Melanie's birth scene in
Gone with the Wind is typical of the way literature and films
stress how unladylike it is to lose control during labor.
Such expressions of pain conflict with the images middle-
class women have of themselves. Groans, cries, and other
noises also make the labor staff uncomfortable. With the
kindest of intentions, they rush to "rescue" the mother,
by offering pain-relieving drugs, or to coach her out of
letting go with breathing patterns. Birth is a time when
even the most independent woman really needs support.
Supportive attendants will allow the mother to express her
feelings. Support can sometimes be as simple as acknowledging a mother's exclamation of "Hell, this hurts" with
"Yes, I know," instead of trying to talk her out of her
experience or telling her the labor will get worse. Pain may
be the only way that some women feel they can communicate their deep need for support at this time, and the
message will be missed if rescue measures are employed.

Beneath a woman's fear of doing "poorly" in labor lie
her fears of pain, genital mutilation, and loss of self-esteem. All these fears are linked with a person's fear of
death. Birth brings forth life but involves confrontation
with the thought of death. Although extremely rare
among healthy women in affluent societies, it is possible
for a woman to die in childbirth. Fears of death — of
mother or child — are submerged, rarely verbalized.
However, these fears may be revealed in a woman who
makes no preparation, emotional or physical, for her
baby's arrival.

Psychologist Leni Schwartz worked with pregnant couples over many months while researching her book *The
World of the Unborn*. Compiling her data, she was struck by
how accurately each couple, within an ongoing support
group stressing feelings and emotions, was able to predict
the outcome of their births. Schwartz found that feelings
offer great potential for learning, as they provide the true

basis on which greater understanding of ourselves can develop.

Letting Go

The notion of control is a polarized concept that inevitably brings to mind its antithesis — loss of control. Most childbirth preparation promises a control that can never be realized because of the nature of birth. When the body starts to take over, the person's first line of attack is usually to attempt more control. This never seems to work, whether the object of control is a speech defect, an unruly teenager, or a labor contraction. The paradox demonstrates the law of reversed effort. The harder we try to fall asleep, to remember a name, to have an orgasm, or to become pregnant, the more it seems to escape us. Yet when we give up, what we seek may happen easily.

Letting go in any way can seem very frightening because we fear that we will fall apart. Loss of control is one of the deepest "falling anxieties" in the human psyche. Newborn babies demonstrate fear of falling if support is rapidly withdrawn from them. This is a survival mechanism. In childhood, to fall down or to fall behind others walking ahead is associated with feelings of failure. Loss of support, not being physically grounded, means loss of contact with reality and one's feelings. People who are afraid of their bodies are also afraid of falling, of letting go.

Individual adjustment to personal crisis depends not only on a person's accepting that the unexpected will happen but also on his or her being able to let go — of the past, of old beliefs, strategies, and rationalizations that are no longer appropriate. The law of causality does not apply in life or in labor, as all the variables affecting human behavior can never be known or controlled. Nothing is absolutely safe. We can only explore our unique paths of adult growth if we free ourselves to flow with whatever our lives have to offer.

Letting go means living in the present. Ambitions lie in the future and fear of failure is based on past experience.

Every act of birth requires the courage to let go of something, to let go of the breast, to let go of the lap, to let go of the hand, to let go eventually of all certainties, and to rely on one thing: one's own power to be aware and to respond; that is, one's creativity. To be creative means to consider the whole process of life as a process of birth, and not to take any stage of life as a final stage.
ERICH FROMM

In all . . . activities of mind and body it is essential, if we are to do our work adequately, that we should cultivate an attitude of confidence — confidence in our capacity to do the job and indifference to possible failure.
ALDOUS HUXLEY

More often, we are aware of *not* living in the present. (An example of this that most people have experienced is driving somewhere and reaching a destination without being aware of any landmark on the way.) This isolation from the world is carried to a deliberate extreme by people who wear portable headsets to jog, cycle, or commute.

Living in the present does not mean that we should avoid setting goals, but that we should choose goals that reflect our present needs, changing them as our priorities shift. Goals invested with personal significance can become part of the process of living. The achievement is less important than the adventure and pleasure we derive from following a path that is optimal for our own needs.

Letting go cannot be taught. It is gained — or rather regained — from early childhood. When a child learns to walk or talk, he or she tries and tries again, but does not use force or ambition. We can learn from children that effort diminishes awareness; sensitivity is a more fruitful approach. Development of a child is based on sensation and movement, a combination of feeling and response that begins in the mother's uterus. Later scholastic learning takes over from organic learning. Lessons and examinations become the priority in formal education, despite the fact that people learn better in more flexible ways. This has been pointed out by reform teachers such as John Holt and A. S. Neill, who recognized that people are ruled more by their emotions than their intellects.

The Importance of Prenatal Bonding

Pregnancy is a marvelous manifestation of the ever-shifting universe. It is a living, changing experience, both spiritual and physical, linking each pregnant woman with the regeneration of all life forms. An obviously pregnant woman attracts friendly inquiries and confidences from total strangers.* Their interest and approval provides so-

* This is only a recent state of liberation for pregnant women. Victorians were ashamed to go out on the street and hid themselves, giving rise to the term *confinement*, which is still in use today. The colloquial Spanish word for pregnancy is *embarazo*.

cial support for the woman's rite of passage — her transition from lover to mother, from child to parent.

Pregnancy also brings into question how comfortably a woman lives within her body. Helping women to feel positive about being pregnant should be a major goal in early prenatal classes. The more pregnant women appreciate their changing bodies, the more they will trust the forces of nature during labor. Women often grow up seeking ever-more beautiful faces and bodies. They find something wrong with their noses, breasts, legs, hips, or other parts of their anatomies, thanks to society's quest for the perfect female body. Pregnancy is always a vulnerable time and many women feel ugly and resent what a baby is "doing" to their figures. Such women hide their pregnancies under voluminous maternity smocks and would never reveal their enlarging shapes in a bikini or leotard. Early prenatal exercise classes provide a perfect opportunity for expectant mothers to confront and cast off negative self-images and conflicts over pregnancy.

Fear is linked with ambition, fear of the unknown and the fear that I won't like what I'll see when I look at myself.
JOEL KRAMER

A pregnant woman's self-image is often damaged by thoughtless medical attendants. However, remarks that appear to be demeaning can be turned about by a confident pregnant woman so that little damage is done to her self-esteem. For example, *small pelvis* is a term doctors use to refer to the prospect of a difficult birth. A well-adjusted woman might consider this a simple description of her bony anatomy and use the information to seek favorable positions for her labor and delivery. *Elderly primipara* is a medical expression dependent on sociological trends, which reflects the physician's opinion that a woman is above the desirable age for giving birth. (This limit is constantly moving up as more women postpone childbearing as a matter of choice.) Instead of dwelling on the unlikely obstetric difficulties that this term suggests, older mothers can congratulate themselves on their added maturity and deep commitment to parenthood. *Difficult veins*, a phrase used by medical staff having trouble obtaining blood samples, can be turned around so that the mother views the phrase as just a reflection of staff ineptitude rather than of any inadequacy in her circulatory system.

Bonding with the baby, especially postpartum, has re-

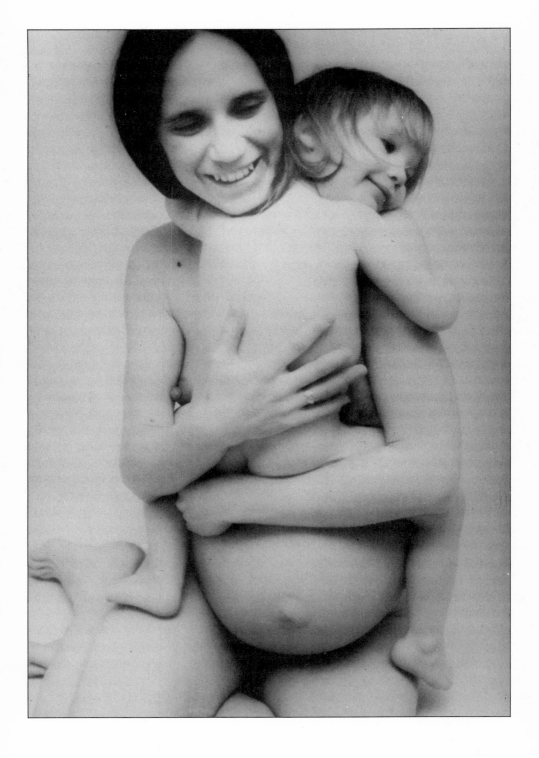

ceived much publicity, but a mother's need to bond with her pregnant body is not really appreciated by most childbirth educators or parents. This is due to a common view of the body as separate and inferior to the mind. Bonding occurs in time, like birth, and is not an isolated event. Some years ago, researchers defined the critical period when parents could fall in love with their newborn as the immediate moments after birth. In studies of premature and caesarean babies, when postpartum parent-infant contact was denied, researchers found that there was increased incidence of maternal rejection of the infant and of later child abuse. These studies have helped to make the hospital birth experience more human and to allow new families privacy together immediately following a birth. Yet in the Netherlands, a stronghold of natural birth (and until recently homebirth) and hospital infant rooming-in, many parents admitted that it took weeks, sometimes months, for them to feel that a newborn really belonged to them. Ideally, then, bonding must begin before birth.

By enhancing physical awareness and pleasure, expectant parents can be creative in expressing enjoyment of pregnancy, birth, and the care of their infant. Couples who spend a lot of time stroking the pregnant abdomen and physically contacting the unborn child continue after birth to touch and caress their baby. Cultures in which infants enjoy much physical closeness with their parents and in which adolescents are given the freedom for sexual experience before marriage show the least incidence of crime and violence. Comfortable sensuality in a child leads to development of healthy adult sexuality with obvious benefits for society.

Dr. Frans Veldman, the founder of Haptonomy, emphasizes that affective, affirmative touch is a vital primary need upon which human emotional life develops. He guides pregnant couples not only to become more aware of their babies as unique and special beings but also to communicate with them in pregnancy to secure a happy parent-infant encounter after birth. Interpreting and responding to the wide range of the baby's moods and movements profoundly cements the parents' emotional attachment. The baby discerns the voice and touch of each parent and learns to anticipate and take part in playful games. The mother learns to harmonize her abdominal and pelvic floor muscles with her uterus, giving the baby freedom and allowing the mother to surrender during labor. Gaining suppleness from "inside out," the pregnant woman and her partner can guide and direct the baby's position with their hands and by the woman's active influence on the uterine muscle tone. As these skills are developed, the mother removes any obstacles in the way of her baby's birth and, in fact, with her partner, actively assists her child during birth by communicating with the infant emotionally and physically throughout the labor.

Many pregnant women are unaware of their babies' sensitivity and their own abilities to invoke a response from their unborn children. One study in Australia in which expectant mothers made sketches of their unborn children revealed that mothers grossly underestimated the development that takes place at each phase of pregnancy and the unborn's human appearance and characteristics.

Even without any knowledge of embryology, many parents spontaneously bond with their babies in utero by naming the baby, singing lullabies, visualizing the infant's sex and features, as well as reacting playfully to fetal movements. Many parents know what kind of music their unborn child prefers and what noises disturb the baby. Some pregnant women sense the emotions behind their babies' movements and can distinguish between kicking as a sign of distress and simple exercise. Certain expectant mothers have keen intuitions about their unborn babies, such as the presence of twins. In the rare cases when something is not quite right with the baby, mothers have usually sensed it.

Medical science acknowledges that maternal observation can play a useful role in counting fetal movements as substitute for complex and technological tests that measure fetal well-being. The rhythms of uterine life are also a key to the unborn child's personality. Psychiatrist Thomas Verny quotes a study indicating that babies who kicked a lot in the uterus grow into anxious children, while quieter babies retain placid natures after birth. Recent research suggests that an unborn baby is not merely a passive passenger during labor but plays a role in the initiation and progress of his or her own birth. Adult recollections about conscious choice in the birth process are detailed in *Life Before Life* by Helen Wambach, Ph.D.

An expectant mother's emotions and activities are known to have a powerful and lasting effect on her baby. Adults who have relived their birth and uterine existence through Primal Therapy, hypnosis, and other regression techniques, report experiences such as attempted abortions, maternal trauma, noxious tastes and sensations, as well as feelings of joy and bliss. Also to be found in the literature are birth memories of small children, who spontaneously supply precise obstetric details relating to their labors and deliveries. Exact comments made by the doctor or nurse, and descriptions of their clothing have also been remembered by children and verified by adults who were present at the births.

It is clear that the creation of a new life can be the most responsible and exciting undertaking in a couple's existence. New dimensions of the pregnancy and birth experience, for both parents and child, are being explored and integrated all the time. Just as the recent revolution in physics and natural science demands a new conceptual framework, so we must look at childbirth and its preparation from a fresh, holistic perspective. The softening of the hard sciences has shown that riddles about life are not solved by applying mechanical principles that served scientists well in the past. Likewise, birth is not a problem to be solved by the application of more and more technology. Rather, a philosophical overhaul of childbirth preparation is needed so that parents and professionals will value the broadest human qualities of childbearing and let themselves be guided by feelings, intuitions, and insights, thus honoring the wisdom of each individual's body, mind, and spirit.

The life of an individual is the life of his body. Since the living body includes the mind, the spirit and the soul, to live the life of the body is to be mindful, spiritual and soulful.
ALEXANDER LOWEN

Resources

Books and Articles

THE UNIVERSE IN CONSTANT FLUX

Capra, Fritjof. *The Tao of Physics*. New York: Bantam, 1975. A pioneering book that integrates modern science and Eastern mysticism.

MEDICINE — HOLISTIC AND MECHANICAL

Bursztajn, Harold, M.D., Richard I. Feinbloom, M.D., Robert M. Hamm, Ph.D., and Archie Brodsky. *Medical Choices, Medical Chances: How Patients, Families and Physicians Can Cope with Uncertainty*. New York: Merloyd Lawrence, 1981. Contrasts mechanistic and holistic perspectives in decision-making; detailed case histories of birth and death.

Cousins, Norman. *Anatomy of an Illness*. New York: Bantam, 1979. One man's successful battle against a severe joint disease with vitamin C and laughter.

Mehl, Lewis E. *Mind and Matter: Foundation for Holistic Health*, Volume 1. Berkeley, Calif.: Mindbody Press, 1981. Practical approaches and case histories set in a broad conceptual framework.

Mendelsohn, Robert S., M.D. *Confessions of a Medical Heretic*. New York: Warner, 1979. A caustic and witty attack on the "religion" of medicine and its conventional procedures such as lab tests, x-rays, immunization, and the annual physical checkup.

ADULT GROWTH

Gould, Roger. *Transformations*. New York: Simon and Schuster, 1978. Overcoming the illusion of safety in adult life and developing freedom and autonomy.

Sheehy, Gail. *Passages: Predictable Crises of Adult Life*. New York: Bantam, 1977. An entertaining book dealing with stages of personal development in adults.

PHILOSOPHY

Kramer, Joel. *The Passionate Mind: A Manual for Creatively Living with One's Self*. Millbrae, Calif.: Celestial Arts, 1974. A simple and direct discussion of fundamental questions such as belief, freedom, fear, time, sexuality, and love.

Pirsig, Robert. *Zen and the Art of Motorcycle Maintenance.* New York: Bantam, 1975. A father and son explore the meaning of life on a cross-country trip. A very readable, informal presentation of philosophical traditions.

Watts, Alan. *Nature, Man and Woman.* New York: Random House, 1970. An inspiring examination of the human place in the universe and the relationship between the sexes. Explores the art of feeling, sexuality, ecstasy, spirituality, and love.

————. *The Wisdom of Insecurity.* New York: Random House, 1951. An invaluable message for an age of anxiety, stressing awareness, insight, the wisdom of the body, and living in the present.

FAMILY RELATIONSHIPS

Friday, Nancy. *My Mother, My Self.* New York: Dell, 1978. A penetrating and absorbing book dealing with all levels of mother-daughter relationships.

Janov, Arthur. *The Feeling Child.* New York: Simon and Schuster, 1975. The importance of freedom and acceptance in the development of a child's "real" self. How to avoid inducing fear, tension, conflict, and neuroses in children.

Liedloff, Jean. *The Continuum Concept.* New York: Warner, 1972. How children are happier, more relaxed, and more independent in cultures where they experience much body contact and share adult lives — always present but never the center of adult attention.

Prescott, James W. "Body Pleasure and the Origins of Violence," *Bulletin of the Atomic Scientists,* November 1975. A neuropsychologist contends that the greatest threat to world peace comes from those nations that have the most depriving environments for their children and that are most repressive of sexual expression and female sexuality.

LOVE

Fromm, Erich. *The Art of Loving: An Enquiry into the Nature of Love.* New York: Harper and Row, 1965. A cultural, philosophical, and psychological discussion of the value and expression of love.

Jampolsky, Gerald G., M.D. *Love Is Letting Go of Fear.* New York: Bantam, 1981. A short, illustrated handbook with tips for personal transformation. Deals with anger, forgiveness, living in the past, and self-responsibility.

LEARNING VERSUS EDUCATION

Holt, John. *How Children Learn*. New York: Dell, 1967. The founder of *Growing Without Schooling* (a parents' resource and support network at 729 Boylston Street, Boston, MA 02116) shows how conventional education is ineffective and degrading. Describes how children figure out the world for themselves through play and motivation.

Neill, A. S. *Summerhill: A Radical Approach to Child Rearing*. New York: Pocket, 1977. Observations of a pioneering British educator and original thinker on the needs of children for freedom, responsibility, and creativity.

FEELING AND MOVEMENT

Janov, Arthur. *The Primal Scream*. New York: G. P. Putnam, 1970. How birth trauma and emotional deprivation in childhood cause neurotic defenses that can be broken down through Primal Therapy so that the real, feeling self emerges.

Lowen, Alexander, M.D. *Bioenergetics*. New York: Penguin, 1975. How the language of the body expresses the problems of the mind. Simple techniques for becoming aware of tension, stress, fear, and anxiety and for releasing negative emotions through body work.

———. *Depression and the Body: The Biological Basis of Faith and Reality*. New York: Penguin, 1972. Explores the universality of depression (and low back pain and myopia) with therapeutic remedies.

PRENATAL BONDING

McGarey, Gladys, M.D. *Born to Live: A Holistic Approach to Childbirth*. Phoenix, Ariz.: Gabriel Press, 1980. A homebirth practitioner shares her insights and unusual experiences with pregnancy and birth. Accounts of miraculous healings and transpersonal experiences.

Schwartz, Leni, Ph.D. *The World of the Unborn: Nurturing Your Child Before Birth*. New York: Richard Marek, 1980. The significance of the baby's prenatal environment and the personal growth of couples through the childbearing experience.

Verny, Thomas, M.D., with John Kelly. *The Secret Life of the Unborn Child*. New York: Summit, 1981. Shows that the unborn child develops a sense of self by the sixth month of pregnancy and that adult personalities and predispositions are shaped from feelings and experiences in the uterine environment. Suggests how positive maternal emotions can have a beneficial influence on the baby.

BIRTH MEMORIES

Grof, Stanislav, M.D. *Realms of the Human Unconscious: Observations from LSD Research.* New York: E. P. Dutton, 1976. An erudite text with fascinating case histories. Perinatal experiences analyzed in a framework of prenatal, labor, birth, and postpartum phases.

Mathison, Linda. "Birth Memories," *Mothering* 21 (Fall 1981). Details of own births spontaneously supplied by children aged two to three.

Wambach, Helen. *Life Before Life.* New York: Bantam, 1979. Amazing recollections of birth and prenatal and past life experiences made by 750 adults under hypnosis.

Film

Tefay, Henry. *Long Ago Hurt.* Available for rental from Maternal and Child Health Center, 2464 Massachusetts Ave., Cambridge, MA 02140. A powerful film made by an Australian Primal therapist showing adults reliving their birth trauma.

Journals

Brain/Mind Bulletin, Marilyn Ferguson, Editor, Interface Press, P.O. Box 42247, Los Angeles, CA 90042. A newsletter published every three weeks on current body-mind research; birth and bonding often featured.

East-West Journal, published by the Kushi Foundation, P.O. Box 1200, Brookline Village, MA 02147. Explores the dynamic equilibrium that unifies apparently opposite values. Many articles on pregnancy and birth; excellent macrobiotic recipes.

Mothering, P.O. Box 2208, Dept. B.L., Albuquerque, NM 87103. A bimonthly magazine dealing with pregnancy, birth, and parenthood. Alternative philosophies, health remedies, and fascinating ads of all kinds of home businesses of interest to families.

New Age Journal, P.O. Box 1200, Allston, MA 02134. A monthly periodical published by Interface (see below) with articles on holistic health. Interesting ads and calendar.

Whole Life Times, 18 Shepard Pl., Brighton, MA 02135. A national newspaper, directory, and calendar, covering health, personal growth, and the environment.

Yoga Journal, 2054 University Ave., Berkeley, CA 94704. Articles on pregnancy, holistic health, and social issues, as well as yoga.

Organizations

American Holistic Medical Association, 6932 Little River Turnpike, Annandale, VA 22003. Referrals to alternative physicians.

Association for Birth Psychology, 444 E. 82nd St., New York, NY 10028. Publishes the quarterly *Birth Psychology Bulletin.* The Elizabeth Fehr Natal Therapy Institute (at the same address) assists people in reexamining birth trauma to relieve anxiety and facilitate insight into the ways people behave.

Feldenkrais Guild, Main Office, P.O. Box 11145, San Francisco, CA 94101. Referrals to certified instructors in the awareness-through-movement approach of Moshe Feldenkrais.

Himalayan International Institute of Yoga Science and Philosophy, P.O. Box 88, Honesdale, PA 18431. Yoga, meditation, psychology, holistic health, nutrition, and Eastern studies. Publishes a free monthly newsletter, the quarterly *Research Bulletin,* and many books. Lectures, workshops, seminars and residential training programs. Also regional branch centers.

Institute for the Alexander Technique, 295 Seventh Ave., New York, NY 10001. Instruction and referrals to practitioners who teach F. Matthias Alexander's approach for increased coordination of mind and body.

Interface, 230 Central St., Newton, MA 02166. Educational programs in holistic health. Variety of reasonably priced lectures and workshops. Higher degrees also offered.

International Polarity Foundation, 511 Main St., Fort Lee, NJ 07024. Information on Polarity therapy and referrals to therapists who work with active and passive touch to balance the body's energy paths.

International Primal Association, 251 W. 89th St., 7B, New York, NY 10024. Listings of Primal therapists who assist clients to get in touch with their feelings through reliving early experiences.

International Society for Research and Development of Haptonomy, Mas Del Ore, 66400 OMS P.O., France. Training, workshops, and publications (in Dutch and French) on the emotional life that evolves from the sense of touch. For information on courses for professional training in the U.S.A., contact: Maternal and Child Health Center, 2464 Massachusetts Avenue, Cambridge, MA 02140.

Radix Institute, P.O. Box 97, Ojai, CA 93023. Certification for teachers in Radix education for feeling and purpose therapy. Workshops, Radix intensives, listings of teachers in the U.S.

Rebirth International, Campbell Hot Springs, P.O. Box 38, Sierraville, CA 96126, and Walton Training Center, 43 Gardiner Pl., Walton, NY 13956. Rebirthing techniques as developed by Leonard Orr, coauthor of *Rebirthing in The New Age* (Millbrae, CA: Celestial Arts, 1977).

Trager Institute, 300 Poplar Ave., Suite 5-Y, Mill Valley, CA 94941. A system of passive and active movements ("Mentastics") developed by Dr. Milton Trager for psychophysical integration. Training appointments and referrals.

CHAPTER 2

Childbirth Education — Its Problems and Potential

People know what they have been taught, but learn little from their own doing. People come to feel that they need to be "educated" . . . Learning thus becomes a commodity, and like any commodity that is marketed, it becomes scarce.
IVAN ILLICH

CLASSES IN prepared childbirth were not available for our grandmothers. Today these classes are a middle-class pursuit, with few exceptions. Much of the impetus for childbirth education has come from obstetrical technology and attempts to explain, criticize, or modify it. Expectant parents look for help from so-called birth experts because nothing in our modern way of life prepares us to experience childbirth. Many couples attend classes to learn what is going to happen to them; others want a magic recipe for a painless labor that fits in with a mechanistic view of the body's role in childbirth.

The Limitations of Childbirth Education

Childbirth education has typically focused on preparation for labor and delivery, and classes occur during the last few weeks of pregnancy. The months before and after birth have been generally overlooked, and the benefits of preventive prenatal measures, such as good nutrition and exercise, are therefore limited. The last trimester of pregnancy is rather late for a couple to confront their beliefs about birth and to open up to the emotional aspects of childbearing.

Fortunately, more early pregnancy and postpartum

groups are emerging. Not only do early prenatal classes provide support and information when they are needed but sessions spaced through pregnancy help a mother defuse her apprehension about the birth day. Classes oriented toward pregnancy include workshops on exercise, health care, and nutrition, as well as a discussion of sexual, physical, and emotional changes. Communication among a woman and her partner and their unborn child is ideally a central focus through the different phases of pregnancy. Each couple's decision about where the birth will take place and choice of attendants is made easier within such a support group.

Childbirth education is geared toward the intellectual functions of the left brain and fosters the belief that women can use their minds to control their bodies and their births if they follow certain prescriptions. For many couples, learning control in childbirth classes is paramount, and they become anxious if the "breathing" is not presented early in the program. Such people also place great store on practice, for repetition comforts the left-brain function that depends on memory. Only an illusion of safety is provided, however, and these couples benefit most from a complete reversal of attitude. No amount of rehearsal will promise a script for birth. Every birth is different. Each labor must run its own course and will, no matter how much control is attempted. Techniques of control merely keep a mother's conscious mind busy in her attempt to push aside both the unknown and the fear of the unknown. The stress of "staying in control" clamps down her body's armor segments (jaw, throat, eyes, pelvis) and prevents her from remaining flexible and rooted in her body.

Paradoxically, what people most need to learn, they cannot be taught or educated to do.
IVAN ILLICH

The English obstetrician Grantly Dick-Read committed himself to the cause of natural, fearless childbirth in the 1930s. His classic *Childbirth Without Fear* is as popular as ever, and reveals this unusual man's insight, compassion, and humility. In contrast, Dr. Fernand Lamaze, working in France, developed a very structured approach based on Pavlovian techniques that he witnessed in Russia. Lamaze also trained *monitrices* (labor coaches) to work as part of

A society that values planned teaching above autonomous learning cannot but teach man to keep his engineered place.
IVAN ILLICH

his team. The teachings of Lamaze became the first and foremost method of organized childbirth preparation, due primarily to promotion by Marjorie Karmel, an American who, in *Thank You, Dr. Lamaze*, wrote about her child's birth in France. The early instigators of the Lamaze method were obliged to offer an academic and controlled educational program to gain acceptance by the medical establishment. Although the philosophy of childbirth preparation has evolved beyond this today, much credit is due to Lamaze programs, which were historically significant in changing childbirth practices. A go with the flow approach would not have been possible in the social climate of the 1950s when births were handled with scopolamine* and general anesthesia. Influence of the less structured Dick-Read method waned until the 1970s when the Read Natural Childbirth Foundation was formed in California to revive the lone pioneer's philosophy. However, over the decades, childbirth educators have generally only modified original Lamaze concepts and techniques or developed alternatives based on left-brain function and separation between mind and body. One example is the method advocated by Robert Bradley, M.D., which is taught by an organization called the American Academy of Husband-Coached Childbirth.

The transformation of learning into education paralyzes man's poetic ability, his power to endow the world with his personal meaning.
IVAN ILLICH

Preparation for childbirth that is based on mechanistic principles frequently cultivates performance anxiety. That is, an expectant mother and her partner must grapple with the likelihood that they may not remember everything they were taught in class, or that they may not have practiced enough, so that the promised control will be lost. Dr. Lamaze warned women, "You will be asked to put forth great efforts . . . a great expenditure of energy . . . and you will succeed — provided you have prepared for it. In that way you will get through; otherwise you will fail." When birth is seen as a performance or a test, then by the same token, there comes a time when all the studying and rehearsing has to be set aside. Every expectant couple just must do their best during labor.

Practice is mechanical and always removes you from what "is."
JOEL KRAMER

* A drug causing loss of memory.

How can birth be subject to ambition or be a mechanically controlled event, like putting people on the moon? Can women be taught how to give birth, how to prepare for labor, and in a classroom? Dr. Lamaze admonished his pregnant clients to be "good students" and told them they were "back on the school benches." Isn't there instinctive knowledge within a mother's nervous system that has passed down through generations? Doesn't the female body that knows how to grow a baby also know how to birth it? Does the mind control the labor or does a woman's body guide her mind, signaling when to work and when to rest? How can couples coordinate their need to control the birth environment, exercising their rights and responsibilities, and at the same time let themselves relax and be led by the labor?

The essence of creativity is an aware balance between control and surrender.
JOEL KRAMER

Although couples undoubtedly enjoy childbirth classes and benefit from them in many ways, conventional prenatal preparation serves hospitals, doctors, and instructors better than they serve expectant couples. Instructors rarely meet a couple's needs for physical and psychological adaptation and instead teach techniques that can actually interfere with the harmony of the birth process. Methods fit in well with a mechanistic view of the world, for more emphasis is placed on classroom learning than on self-exploration. As a result, many couples bury themselves in the labor guidebook and miss the view. After attending one of my workshops, one childbirth educator ruefully commented, "I've had two births with breathing patterns and other distraction techniques, but now I want to have another baby so I can *feel* what giving birth is like."

We live what we know. If we believe the universe and ourselves to be mechanical, we will live mechanically. On the other hand, if we know that we are part of an open universe, we will live more creatively and powerfully.
MARILYN FERGUSON

The Training of Childbirth Educators

Professional childbirth education training is not part of any undergraduate curriculum. It is either learned on the job or through various organizations concerned with a particular method. Certification, group membership, and continuing education encourage instructors to continue with one method to the practical exclusion of others.

Methods are for creating things that do not yet exist.
ALAN WATTS

Lamaze, Dick-Read, and Bradley are household words

to millions of people. These birthing theories were all developed by men and have hardened into competing doctrines for the purpose of training teachers and attracting expectant couples. Since the similarities of the methods are more obvious than their differences, couples have difficulty sorting out various options for "being prepared." All methods vary with the personality of the instructor. Some couples take more than one series to get a varied perspective. There is an enormous amount of often-conflicting information on childbearing, each method promising its own special rewards for rightful participation. Couples tend to become avid supporters of a teacher's techniques. The effectiveness of the method thus becomes a self-fulfilling prophecy.

Our society's increasing regulation and legislation have not overlooked childbirth education. There is ongoing debate over who is eligible to assume the role of childbirth educator. Should instructors be mothers or physicians, nurses, midwives, teachers, physical therapists, or others in the health care field? Childbirth educators generally are trained rather than educated, in the sense of the Latin word *educare*, "to lead out." If a method is to be promulgated, then its curriculum must be made standard. Broad reading on physiology, psychology, or philosophy is not required for certification in childbirth education. Instead, training focuses on current obstetrical practices.

Attending births, surprisingly, is only a minor part of certification requirements. The average childbirth educator is obliged to follow only about half a dozen births. Instructors who do not witness a great variety of women's responses during labor tend to become the conservative core of the movement. They may be more reactionary than the hospital staff they criticize as being unsupportive of an expectant couple's labor techniques. Hospital maternity staff do see the whole range of labors and the different ways that individuals cope with labor, despite what the mothers may have been taught in childbirth classes. Labor-room personnel may be justifiably skeptical of some of the prescriptions given to pregnant couples, especially the more elaborate breathing patterns.

Changing Members of the Birth Team

Childbirth education began much earlier in other English-speaking countries, Europe, and Scandinavia, where traditionally it has been taught by physical therapists working as part of a team with midwives or general practitioners. Until recently, obstetricians in those countries were consulted only when there was an abnormal development during pregnancy or labor. Indeed, there is no Dutch word for the medical specialist who attends a normal labor, as no tradition exists of this in the Netherlands. The Dutch physician who assists a birth with complications is known as a *gynaecoloog* ("gynecologist"), which strictly means "one who deals with *diseases* of women."

Obstetric, *from the* Latin obstare, *"to stand in the way," "stand in front of."* Webster's New Collegiate Dictionary

In the United States, obstetricians took childbirth over from midwives and family practitioners just a few decades ago. The power and influence of American culture have led to this also happening abroad. Increasing use of obstetricians is associated everywhere with high costs and heavy intervention in childbirth, which should not require a medical specialist in more than 10 percent of cases. Of course, there are obstetricians committed to assisting natural childbirth, but generally the outrage expressed by many parents and professionals is justified. Yet the increasing number of exorbitant malpractice suits perpetuates the cycle of defensive medical management.* As parents take back more responsibility for their decisions in labor and birth, the problem of lawsuits should diminish. Most malpractice suits result from lack of communication. Malpractice is more likely to happen with a busy physician than with midwives, who spend more time with the mother prenatally as well as during labor.

Male science disregards female experiences because it can never share them.
GRANTLY DICK-READ

Obstetricians use their status to gain all and give nothing.
GRANTLY DICK-READ

Growing numbers of homelike birth centers across the country have been created in response to consumer pres-

---

* In practicing defensive medicine, physicians order tests and perform procedures "just in case," so that they cannot be held liable for neglecting to do so. Insurance companies fuel this increase in intervention — for example, by reimbursing patients for the cost of procedures but not for counseling.

sure for change and the homebirth movement. These centers may or may not be part of a hospital and are usually staffed by midwives. Birth centers vary greatly in atmosphere and protocol and operate cautiously so as not to risk their existence by alienating the medical establishment. As a result, about one third to one fifth of laboring women are transferred from birth centers to regular hospital labor and delivery units. Generally, out-of-hospital birth centers are more autonomous than those that are part of a hospital. Unfortunately, in many hospitals, the only difference between birth rooms (often there is only one per hospital) and traditional labor and delivery rooms is decor (wallpaper, bedspread, and a few potted plants) — a mere gesture to consumer demands for a homelike birth environment and a holistic approach. Meanwhile, back at the pelvis, business as usual!

Birth rooms are a cop-out. Every woman should have the right to a physiological birth without interference.
DORIS HAIRE

The renaissance of midwifery, which the United States is currently enjoying, has already increased the satisfaction of birth for many women, with no compromise in safety. In many hospitals, such as the North Central Bronx Hospital in New York, the outcome for mothers and babies has actually improved, thanks to the staff midwives' physiological approach to birth. Despite a local high-risk, indigent population, the hospital's birth statistics are as good as those of any private hospital in New York City serving white, middle-class mothers.

The Environment of Childbirth Education

Hospital policies and procedures place a great deal of pressure on childbirth educators, especially those who teach in a hospital or clinic. Hospitals prefer to engage their own maternity staff as instructors to represent the institutional point of view. Rarely do hospitals use consumer advisors in developing a childbirth education program, whereas community-sponsored classes use professional consultants to design classes that serve a couple best. Instructors in hospitals must reassure expectant couples of the desirability and safety of hospital routines and medical interventions during labor, such as the use of intravenous drip, electronic fetal heart monitors, medication, and anesthesia. Since childbirth classes originated in communities, hospital prenatal classes are in almost all cases a duplication, and not an improvement, in service.

The community-based childbirth educator is forced to compete against hospital classes that are often subsidized and that may offer a rebate on a couple's maternity bill. Some hospitals make it difficult for expectant parents attending independent classes to obtain a tour of hospital labor and delivery areas.

Community-based prenatal classes, whether taught by individuals or members of a childbirth group, are more oriented toward the needs of the consumer than hospital classes. The smaller number of couples per class leaves room for sharing. However, instructors in the community cannot afford to discuss obstetric practices in ways that will aggravate local hospitals or obstetricians if they wish to fill their classes. One childbirth educator commented, "Imagine if we told couples how it *really* was . . . perhaps we'd lose fewer teachers from our group." No wonder many of these dedicated and enthusiastic teachers suffer "childbirth preparation burnout." They are caught in a triple bind. If they describe accurately how birth is managed in some hospitals, couples would become very fearful. If expectant parents anticipate a warm and flexible birth environment and find out that such is not the case in the hospital they use, their disappointment is inevitable and bitter. If the instructors advocate childbirth without drugs or anesthesia and these are needed, parents may harbor feelings of guilt and failure.

To thine own self be true.
WILLIAM
SHAKESPEARE

Each instructor must teach what she knows in her bones to be true. A dynamic teacher is constantly changing, becoming more self-aware. At the same time, couples must be warned that almost all hospitals and doctors have expectations based on the mechanical model of birth.

The Influence of Childbirth Education

Lengthy discussions of labor interventions that now form a large part of childbirth preparation can be seen as an indirect endorsement of such interference. The growth of classes that offer preparation for caesarean section (now known as caesarean "birth"), for example, indicates an acceptance of the fact that the caesarean rate has escalated enough to warrant special prenatal preparation. Nancy Cohen, cofounder of the first caesarean support group, now considers caesarean birth preparation in most cases an "insult to women" and dedicates herself to caesarean prevention. Other educators recommend that no mention of labor complications be made in class so as to avoid possible negative effects on expectant parents from such information.

We can compromise for a time, but eventually we realize that ambivalence is like deciding to recognize the law of gravity only sometimes and in certain places.
MARILYN FERGUSON

Most childbirth educators in these dilemmas attempt to take a neutral attitude. Sitting on the fence with regard to the medical management of birth, however, does not help couples evaluate the facts or set priorities. Nor does neutrality adequately support a couple who desires birth without interference. Although there is never any guarantee of a birth's outcome, it is important for expectant parents to make a commitment to birth with no intervention and to receive strong encouragement from like-minded obstetric team members. Natural childbirth implies the freedom for a couple to behave naturally during labor and also implies no interference during labor that may adversely affect its progress.

The term *natural childbirth* causes confusion among both maternity care providers and consumers. Childbirth educators worry that doctors may be annoyed by a term that suggests primitive women squatting on the ground (although this may be the best position for birth!). Since most obstetricians increasingly interfere with labor, they rightly view the term as an inaccurate description of the service they provide. If birth really were natural, why would childbirth preparation programs and learned techniques be necessary? After all, people enjoy food and sexual intercourse without knowing the anatomy and physiology involved in digestion and sexual response.

Natural childbirth means no physical, chemical or psychological condition likely to disturb the normal sequence of events or disrupt the natural phenomenon of parturition.
GRANTLY DICK-READ

The preferred term, unfortunately, has become *prepared childbirth*. This covers every contingency of hospital intervention and accommodates all childbirth education methods. *Prepared childbirth* appeals both to couples who want to "try" (as they often word it) for natural childbirth and those who don't like the associations of *natural* and prefer to go along with medical staff advice and routine hospital procedures. Both the notions of "trying" and *prepared childbirth* allow educators, physicians, and nurses to pretend they are talking about normal birth when in fact they are preparing women for the modern substitute — technology, drugs, and surgery.

All institutions are slow to change because so many people in them must agree on a new direction. In regard to childbirth, it is not simply obstetricians and nurses who decide whether a hospital will, for example, hire midwives, buy double beds, or allow mothers to walk around during labor. Anesthesiologists, pediatricians, and neonatologists voice opinions as well.

Hospitals have been reluctant to make changes based on recommendations made by professional childbirth educators, such as alternative birth positions or nourishment during labor. In the long run, it will be the general public who forces institutional change. Angry parents, not professionals, have gained birth-room access for husbands, cameras, and now siblings. However, couples need to know the influence they can wield, economically, and to be supported by instructors for more freedom during hospital births.

Childbirth educators can help guarantee choices for parents by supporting midwives, homebirth, and alternative birth centers. Community classes in which couples have chosen a variety of maternity care providers and places for birth help to foster public awareness of available options. As consumer advocates, childbirth educators can use their influence to speak out against unnecessary birth interventions and support women seeking normal low-key births.

New Possibilities for Childbirth Education

Preparation for birth should be broadened to encompass a preventive role in screening and resolving physical and psychological problems in pregnancy. Bonding within a family ideally begins long before birth and a joyful preg-

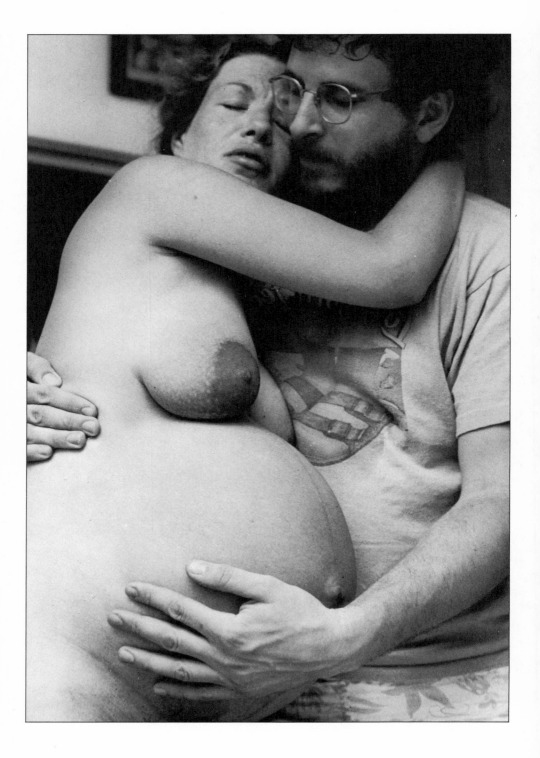

nancy is an excellent foundation for it. Early pregnancy classes offer couples the chance to explore ambivalent feelings, conflicts, aches, nausea, and other difficulties through advice, group support, and appropriate referrals.

It is essential that the expectant mother does not see her body as her enemy or the baby inside as a troublemaker. If a prospective mother feels negative or indifferent toward her pregnancy, then her body will become increasingly strange and unfamiliar to her. The thought of her labor will be especially frightening. Nine months of pregnancy provide a perfect time for developing awareness of body and mind and for personal growth, while also preparing a woman for a creative, natural birth and a strong mother-infant bond.

At the Maternal and Child Health Center in Cambridge, Massachusetts, we offer ongoing prenatal exercise classes, starting as early as possible, even before pregnancy. As the women move and stretch together in class, much information is informally exchanged and absorbed. Meeting several times a week, our groups also offer support for sharing feelings, dreams, and emotions. Many mothers claim that their most significant preparation occurred in those exercise and relaxation classes, and that they felt such a foundation to be more solid than any short course designed for birth preparation in the last trimester.*

The continuum of the childbearing year is also very important. Our center's three-month mother and baby program provides exercise, information, and support for new mothers. Just as pregnant women need to take back responsibility for their births from obstetricians, so mothers need to take back responsibility for their babies from pediatricians. These classes, in which mothers and babies enjoy dancing, exercises, massage, and social interaction, are most helpful in building parental confidence.

Childbirth classes ideally help husbands and other support persons to understand the process of labor and to assist the expectant mother to change her fear of the un-

I can learn from others, but it is only by being in touch with what is going on inside of me that I can see if other points of view make sense for my life.
JOEL KRAMER

* Our childbirth classes for couples consist of three sessions in the first trimester, dealing with pregnancy; three classes in the third trimester, dealing with birth; and a postpartum reunion of the class group.

known to strong self-confidence, while remaining flexible enough to adapt to the unexpected. The striking feature of labor is its variability. Instead of placing their belief in methods, couples need to put their faith in their own resources and inner strength so that they can respond to whatever their particular birth experience will present. This is the way in which every birth is unique and it is both a duty and a privilege for all those who assist birthing women to support their expression of their own individuality. Clearly, no behavior control is appropriate nor will any single model of brand-name techniques do.

Childbirth educators and expectant couples can become enlightened, literally and figuratively, if educators emphasize simple truths and guiding principles, teaching less but allowing the couples to learn more from themselves. It is more important for instructors to help couples articulate questions than to demand certain answers or behavioral responses. Teachers don't need to worry about filling their course curriculum if they delete breathing patterns and structured reactions. Instead, they can be more free to intuit unspoken needs and conflicts in the couples. The quality of childbirth education, like any guided growth process, depends not on the academic qualifications of the instructor but rather on the extent to which that individual is in touch with his or her *self*. Then, he or she can be in touch with others. An educator needs to explore his or her own values, motivations, and deep feelings, because change must occur in oneself before one can evoke change in others. As Wilhelm Reich noted, people need to be wooed out of their armored shells. This is a different process with every person.

The teacher's authority rests on personal liberation. One follows qualities, not people.
MARILYN FERGUSON

Any guidance of breathing, relaxation, awareness, or energy flow must respect normal physiology and facilitate rather than suppress the mother's feelings and emotions. When the holistic unity of mind and body is truly acknowledged, childbirth education can be broadened in many dimensions. This does not mean that childbirth educators should merely fit a new idea here and there into their existing program, but rather that a whole different perspective will dawn on them when they are ready to receive it. It is rather like "seeing" the point of a joke, which is missed if one tries to figure it out. Likewise, if a pregnant woman needs to ask, for example, what *others* think about her planning a homebirth, it strongly suggests that she should not have her baby at home. When both her body and mind are in harmony, a pregnant woman has confidence in her own decision, and she is ready to accept responsibility for the birth's outcome.

Childbirth educators must tell pregnant couples the whole truth about birth. The hard work of labor, pain, and the unpredictable course of birth must be presented so that couples do not resist their bodies but shape realistic expectations of their own resources as they journey into the unknown. A woman must realize that during birth she *is* her labor; she *is* her pain. Instructors must not be afraid to provide evidence against medical or hospital procedures (such as ultrasound, fetal monitoring, drugs, anesthesia, episiotomy), in spite of the risk of causing guilt among mothers who may undergo them.

Many childbirth educators won't talk about pain. They describe labor and birth through rose-colored spectacles. These childbirth educators themselves have not come to terms with the reality of birth.
DIONY YOUNG

Childbirth education in the 1980s is at the crossroads. Much has been achieved since Marjorie Karmel and Elisabeth Bing introduced the Lamaze method of childbirth preparation over thirty years ago. Childbirth education has been associated with improved birth outcome and fewer drugs and complications. However, there are still too many instruments, machines, tubes, and drugs, and the caesarean rate continues to rise among prepared couples.

Medical technology is an increasing threat, with more hazards for the many low-risk mothers than benefits for the few high-risk mothers for whom the technology was designed. Educators must continue to push for more freedom in birthing and more respect for normalcy. Most of all they must be careful not to set themselves up as experts and thus undermine the special power over birth that pregnant women possess.

Resources

Books and Articles

WOMEN AND THE MEDICAL MYSTIQUE

Arms, Suzanne. *Immaculate Deception: A New Look at Childbirth in America.* Boston: Houghton Mifflin, 1975. Describes how hospitals complicate childbirth, compares birth practices in other countries and presents a strong argument for midwifery and homebirth.

Corea, Gena. *The Hidden Malpractice: How Medicine Mistreats Women.* New York: Jove, 1978. A feminist view of medical history's prejudices against women as both consumers and providers of health care.

Mendelsohn, Robert S., M.D. *Mal(e) Practice: How Doctors Manipulate Women.* Chicago: Contemporary Books, 1981. A caustic exposé of common, unnecessary, and harmful medical practices in obstetrics and gynecology.

Scully, Diana. *Men Who Control Women's Health: The Education of Obstetricians and Gynecologists.* Boston: Houghton Mifflin, 1980. A sociologist who followed residents in training describes how obstetricians come to see themselves as surgical specialists while their female clients expect them to be preventive and primary health care practitioners.

MIDWIFERY

Gaskin, Ina May. *Spiritual Midwifery.* Revised Edition. Summertown, Tenn.: Book Publishing Company, 1982. Personal accounts by couples of their midwife-attended births on The Farm, an alternative community. Very good technical and reference sections.

Haire, Doris. "Improving the Outcome of Pregnancy Through Increased Utilization of Midwives," *Journal of Nurse-Midwifery* 26:1 (January/February 1981). A description of the excellent outcome for mothers and babies through midwifery skills, at a hospital in a sociologically depressed area of New York City.

CHILDBIRTH OPTIONS

Bean, Constance. *Methods of Childbirth.* Second Edition, Revised. New York: Doubleday, 1982. Describes different types of preparation for birth. (Skip the controlled breathing.) Good information on hospital procedures and interventions and how to avoid them.

Feldman, Silvia, Ph.D. *Choices in Childbirth*. New York: Bantam, 1980. A "yellow pages" dealing with home and hospital birth, birth centers, breastfeeding, caesareans and community support.

Parfitt, Rebecca. *The Birth Primer: A Source of Traditional and Alternative Methods in Labor and Delivery*. Philadelphia: Running Press, 1977. A thorough guide for options in childbirth preparation.

Organizations

The American Academy of Husband-Coached Childbirth, P.O. Box 5224, Sherman Oaks, CA 91413. Bradley method of preparation.

American College of Home Obstetrics, c/o Gregory White, M.D., 2821 Rose St., Franklin Park, IL 60131. Physicians assisting at homebirths.

American College of Nurse-Midwives, 1012 14th St. N.W., Washington, DC 20005. Professional association of midwives.

American Foundation for Maternal and Child Health, Inc., 30 Beekman Pl., New York, NY 10022. Information and resources.

American Society for Psychoprophylaxis in Obstetrics (ASPO), 1411 K St. N.W., Suite 200, Washington, DC 20005. Lamaze method of preparation.

Association for Childbirth at Home International, Box 1219, Cerritos, CA 90701. Nationwide referrals.

The Birth Place Resource Center, 681 Oak Drive, Menlo Park, CA 94025.

Holistic Childbirth Institute, 1627 Tenth Ave., San Francisco, CA 94112. Alternative approaches to childbirth preparation.

Informed Homebirth, 1811 Burns St., Detroit, MI 48214. Nationwide referrals.

International Association of Parents and Professionals for Safe Alternatives in Childbirth (IAPPSAC), P.O. Box 267, Marble Hill, MO 63764. Publishes a newsletter, the *Directory of Alternative Birth Services*, and the proceedings from their 1976, 1977, and 1978 conferences.

International Childbirth Education Association (ICEA), P.O. Box 20048, Minneapolis, MN 55420. Umbrella organization providing information on all aspects of pregnancy, birth, and parenthood, with a specialized mail-order Bookcenter.

Maternal and Child Health Center, 2464 Massachusetts Ave., Cambridge, MA 02140. A resource center for pregnancy, birth, and postpartum. Classes in prenatal and postpartum exercise, preparation for natural childbirth, parenthood, mothers and infants. Library, referrals, labor support, and individual counseling and therapy.

Midwives Alliance of North America (MANA), % Ina May Gaskin, 156 Drakes La., Summertown, TN 38483.

Obstetrics and Gynecology Section, American Physical Therapy Association, 1156 15th St., N.W., Washington, DC 20005. Referrals to physical therapists specializing in obstetrics and gynecology.

Read Natural Childbirth Foundation, 13301 S. Eliseo Dr., Suite 102, Greenbrae, CA 94904. The Grantly Dick-Read method of prepared childbirth.

Vaginal Birth After Caesarean (VBAC), 10 Great Plain Terr., Needham, MA 02192. For information send stamped, self-addressed envelope and $1 % Nancy Cohen.

CHAPTER 3

A Fresh Look
at Old Techniques

ALTHOUGH women have been giving birth since time began, the lack of cumulative female knowledge and sharing in our society has led us to seek information about birth in books and classes rather than from the native wisdom of community experience. Not so long ago, certificates were routinely awarded to expectant couples on completion of a prepared childbirth series, and there are still hospitals that require these papers if a husband is to be allowed to join his wife for the birth.

Having examined the assumptions on which methods of birth-pain control are based, we will now look at the specific tools of labor management, such as coaching, conditioned response, dissociation, distraction, concentration, focusing, conscious release, and controlled breathing. These mechanical features of childbirth preparation have been developed in the belief that their practice will bring about the desired response in labor. Taught with the best of intentions, this array of behavior control is nevertheless questionable for physical and psychological reasons.

*Formulae are for those
who sidestep the
challenge of new
experience.*
ALAN WATTS

Coaching and the Classroom

Through childbirth education, the status of the accompanying husband has been upgraded to that of coach. The word is convenient to use in class where not all partners are husbands. However, the term *coach* evokes images of organized sports, teams, and captains. It reflects an underlying belief that the natural event of birth is a game to be played, with rules to be followed, behavior to be learned, and appropriate rewards to be received. In the space of just a few weeks, the partner is supposed to become expert and confident in his or her ability to evaluate, prompt, or direct a laboring woman. Not all partners make suitable coaches. A father, especially, is often not able to act as an advocate for his wife and child in the hospital environment. Therefore, some couples prefer to engage the services of a support person who has had experience at births and who can be assertive in the hospital situation.

Practice is usually stressed in most childbirth classes. If a laboring woman experiences difficulty "controlling" her contractions, the staff may comment that she did not practice enough. Skills develop if we regularly rehearse with our voluntary muscles. Training can also occur with involuntary systems, such as lowering blood pressure through meditation. But the value and appropriateness of mechanical practice of classroom techniques designed for a reflex, involuntary experience such as labor need to be examined.

Techniques of Control

Our futile effort at control impedes the flow we might otherwise have in our lives. Once we get out of our own way, we can become ourselves.
MARILYN FERGUSON

The foundation of childbirth education has traditionally been the instructors' concern for psychological control. The expectant mother's mind is the chief weapon in the struggle. Indeed, the term for the best-known type of preparation is *psychoprophylaxis*, which means "mind prevention." Practiced response to commands, concentration, focusing her eyes, and complex breathing patterns occupy what Lamaze called the "cerebral machinery." In this way a laboring woman will try to dissociate her mind from her body to gain control over painful contractions. Lamaze's disciple, Dr. Pierre Vellay, author of *Childbirth Without Pain*, writes, "Like expert engineers with perfect machines and carefully presented information [women] control, direct and regulate their bodies." To these male physicians, giving birth is not like learning to walk, which is preprogrammed and happens without instruction when the individual is physiologically ready. Dr. Lamaze wrote, "A woman must learn how to give birth in the same way that she learns how to swim or write or read." Dr. Vellay advised that a mother "must insist on being trained in the proper way." Because these prominent obstetricians held typically mechanistic views, pregnant women are commonly seen as machines that can be regulated. Dr. Lamaze actually stated that "as the obstetrician is the only one conversant with the dynamic nature of the uterus, he alone can decide how such a labor is progressing"!

Lamaze believed that "speech is the best means we have to prepare women for childbirth." Vellay wrote, "Words by their direct meaning enable the human being to have precise and complex stereotypes, far superior to those formed by the animal through direct signals." The key words are *without pain*. Birthing experts promised pain relief through words ("verbal analgesia"), following psychoprophylactic instruction.

In contrast, it can be argued that "direct signals" are more immediate and powerful than any "instrument of language" during the birth experience. Words, abstract symbols, can be interpreted very differently. Many women have faithfully believed the words of Lamaze but they experienced pain nonetheless.

Methods of childbirth preparation such as Dick-Read and Bradley allow the laboring woman more association with her body and feelings than other methods, but they are much smaller and less influential than the Lamaze organizations. Almost all methods offer instruction drawing on basic techniques for mind control.

Consciousness is seen as an act of restraint. Shame accompanies the failure of restraint, such as crying or blushing.
ALAN WATTS

Society is our extended mind and body. We copy emotions, language and ideas.
ALAN WATTS

Conditioned Response

Psychoprophylaxis is based on classical conditioning (Pavlovian reflexes) and operant, or instrumental, conditioning (as in the behavioral school of psychology popularized by

B. F. Skinner). Training is accomplished with an expectant couple's repetition of the proper words and techniques. These skills supposedly become so automatic to her that in labor the real contraction can be easily displaced, like Pavlov's dog who learned to salivate at the sound of a bell. The promise of an easy, painless, or brief labor is a strong incentive for a woman to practice breathing patterns and other control mechanisms taught in class. Her behavior is thus conditioned to operate for an anticipated reward. Negative reinforcement also operates. If a woman does not follow the method, her labor will surely be painful and the attending medical staff will disapprove of her lack of commitment to her birth method. As Dr. Lamaze wrote, "[A mother's] mind carefully educated, steadfast and alert, will know how to abolish pain. In the same way, it can magnify pain if misfortune and negligence decree that she should fail in her task."

Dissociation and Distraction

All our psychological defenses against suffering are useless. The more we defend, the more we suffer and defending is itself suffering . . . We must give in . . . [Therein] the whole experience of suffering undergoes a startling change.
ALAN WATTS

In childbirth classes, a woman learns to shut out messages from her pregnant body and, through distraction techniques, to keep tight control of her responses. At the same time she is supposed to remain relaxed and apart from her labor contractions. These techniques operate on the premise that if a woman's mind is sufficiently occupied it won't register the pain of labor. In Dr. Lamaze's words, "Training the brain to establish a focus of activity to inhibit awareness from the uterus enables a woman to rule her labor." Distraction is provided by focusing the eyes on one point and performing often elaborate breathing patterns that demand concentration.

Distraction and dissociation are based on the mistaken gap between body and mind, as in the statement "a football player may notice an injury only after the game, because his mind was so occupied at the time that he didn't feel it." Spontaneous participation in a sport is a unified experience of living in the present, totally unlike the structured mechanistic birthing where a woman's mind attempts to control her laboring body. Pain is all a matter of degree and is relieved more by relaxation than control. Individuals vary greatly in the way they interpret and respond to pain. While some athletes don't "notice" an injury, others are carried off the field on stretchers. Likewise there are women in labor who also find their pain unbearable.

Most marathoners run according to the principle of dissociation, although recent literature on the experience of running calls for the opposite approach. The actual winners of marathons discard the philosophy of dissociation and tune in to their bodies. Instead of ignoring or forcing through their pain, such runners meet pain with acceptance and surrender, adjusting their pace and speed to it.

We can filter reality to suit our level of courage. At every crossroads we make the choice again for greater or lesser awareness.
MARILYN FERGUSON

Human experience continuously shifts between the body and mind. While concentrating intently, we may notice that one leg has gone to sleep. There comes a moment when the message from a compressed nerve surpasses the best distraction and any hope for dissociation. When the body demands action, we have to give in and free the leg. At other times, the mind can gently ease the body through its resistance in sport or exercise.

Dissociation may work briefly as a pain-control technique, but it consumes rather than conserves energy. Presented as a condition for feeling less pain, it is similar to conditional love from a parent. Such requirements cause a split between the emotions (which are felt in the body) and conscious thought in order to please an authority.

Concentration

A baby never has to be made to concentrate; he or she is naturally self-composed and effortlessly aware in what pediatricians have termed "the quiet alert state." Many adults want to rediscover this quality of attention, which is usually distorted by our beliefs and attitudes. Heightened awareness occurs spontaneously when an adult's conscious thoughts are released.

In childbirth preparation, the expectant mother is taught

Concentration involves effort, a narrowing of the spectrum of awareness. Concentration strengthens thought and the separation between the concentrator and the concentration.
JOEL KRAMER

to concentrate on breathing patterns and a visual focal point. But the law of reversed effort dictates that no one manages to concentrate intently by sheer will power. When one is interested, concentration occurs naturally.

Focusing

In the context of "new age" therapies, focusing means becoming aware of inner states and feelings, centering oneself. In childbirth education it has an opposite meaning and refers to the technique of visual focusing as a way of distracting a laboring mother's attention to avoid her becoming aware of what is going on in her body.

The strained stares of a pregnant woman rehearsing her focusing skills for labor are far removed from the shining, tranquil eyes of a centered infant. In labor, women may prefer to close their eyes, rather than to focus their vision externally. They find that it is in fact more relaxing for them to tune in to their bodies. Other women find that they can better stay in the present with their eyes open. It is easier to let the eye make natural random movements, such as scanning and blinking, than to stare fixedly at one point. In his classic *The Art of Seeing*, Aldous Huxley describes how forcing the eyes to fix on a point interferes with body relaxation and respiration. The strain leads to shallow, suspended breathing and it is tiring to repress natural bodily movement, however small. While eye contact between a laboring woman and her attendant or partner is helpful for communication, if it is maintained for prolonged periods, it can become forced and mechanical.

Conscious Release

Conscious release, a common technique for relaxation instruction in childbirth classes, is based on the assumption that the mind can relax specific parts of the body by a direct reduction in muscle tension. Two neurological problems inhibit this theory. First, the brain does not know individual muscles, only movements. Second, there are no nerve pathways reaching the conscious brain that register muscle tension. Circuits operate instead at lower levels of the nervous system. A person's natural physiological re-action when asked to relax a specific muscle is to fidget, because movement does reach the conscious brain. Only with biofeedback equipment are tension levels in muscles electronically recorded and supplied to the mind in the form of a visual or auditory signal.

Selective relaxation is another childbirth class technique for practicing dissociation from the physical sensations of labor. For example, one arm is tensed while the rest of the body is kept relaxed. This exercise is repeated with various combinations of limbs simultaneously tensed and relaxed. Expectant couples may have fun checking each other for relaxation during these exercises, but they often rightly question the relevance of this exercise to labor, when in-voluntary muscles will be working. Every movement, however subtle, involves the whole individual. Relaxation on command is mistakenly based on the nonexistent split between a person's body and mind.

Breathing Patterns

Breathing is both a voluntary and involuntary function. Unlike other inner metabolic activities, we can choose to become aware of our breathing at any time. Sensitive to physical and psychological changes, breathing mirrors our emotions. Thus, almost every human potential movement experiments with breath awareness. Breathing indicates our degree of physical exertion and the way we use our energy. Blocking the breath holds back energy, whereas breathing freely and fully lets it flow through the body.

Research by the International Society for Research and Development in Haptonomy discovered that there are consistent respiratory patterns for different psychological states, such as aggression and inner- or outer-directed ac-tivity. Interesting graphs have been made documenting spontaneous breath changes of students doing exams, people in arguments, and people listening to music.

Pacing respiration through deliberate breathing patterns

is common to almost all childbirth preparation methods. The most complex forms of breath control have been found in Lamaze, or psychoprophylactic, training. Dr. Lamaze stated that "respiratory exercises must be directed and controlled carefully and none should be done without medical direction." However, childbirth education has evolved into a paramedical activity, and a mother's breathing techniques are of little interest to obstetricians. These days, the job of monitoring the mother's breathing is given to the birth coach, along with a chart that outlines the different phases of labor with appropriate breathing patterns — such as *choo-choo, hoo-ha*, panting and blowing combinations, "spiral staircase" breathing, or sheep's or butterfly breaths. (One can't help but ask, what is wrong with normal human breathing!) As contractions become more intense, the mother is supposed to do more elaborate breathing patterns for their distraction value. However, with the progress of labor and increase in pain, the mother naturally fatigues.

The use of artificial breathing patterns in labor has been taken for granted by most childbirth educators. Many reasons have been given for teaching a mother to alter this vital and sensitive body process. Whether patterns taught are fast or slow, shallow or deep, plateau or accelerated, instructors have claimed all sorts of positive results — increased oxygenation, distraction from the labor, conditioned response, improved relaxation, and pain relief. The virtues of one breathing pattern over another are debated from time to time, and many educators have greatly modified their breath control techniques. Very few of them, however, have thought to question the principle of controlled breathing in the first place. This is reminiscent of controversy in obstetrics over episiotomy, when physicians debate the type of incision without ever questioning the *need* for surgery.

Doris Haire, president of the American Foundation for Maternal and Child Health, is one of many who have expressed concern about the physiological effects of controlled breathing on a woman in labor. Pregnancy naturally alters maternal respiration; the work of breathing is increased. A woman entering labor breathes differently from a woman who is not pregnant. Although Lamaze claimed that shallow and quick breathing helps the oxygenation of the blood (which it does not), by the third trimester, 99 percent of oxygen is normally present in the circulation. Therefore, rapid panting is not indicated and may in fact lead to disturbance of blood gases.

Expectant couples have been led to believe that "doing the breathing" is their key to a comfortable birth. If a prenatal class is missed or the due date brought forward, some women become anxious that they will not have enough time to learn all the magic breathing patterns. Those in the helping professions are only too flattered to encourage these misconceptions by stressing the importance of breath control. Yet many instructors have confided in me that they found it difficult or even impossible to keep up artificial breathing in their own labors. But they did not value their firsthand experience and they continue to teach the method to their couples. One educator remarked, "Now I know I *did* have a good labor and birth — I breathed in my *own* natural way."

It can be necessary to direct a person's breathing, for example, in lung disease or even during labor if a woman becomes faint from overbreathing. At other times the respiratory system simply takes care of itself. It is illuminating to have a group count the number of breaths they take in a minute to observe the great variation among individuals. The members of the group can observe in each other the difference in how people breathe and where the movement occurs. It goes against physiology to train a woman to abandon her normal breathing responses. Moreover, any externally directed influence on a laboring woman's breathing is undesirable because of the close relationship between breathing and emotions. Many couples today, especially those expecting second babies, seek classes that do not teach artificial breathing — or any other technique of control.

The more you are you the fuller breathflow flows.
PAUL REPS

Inhibiting the Diaphragm

The diaphragm, a major muscle of respiration, separates the chest from the abdomen. Breathing patterns traditionally emphasize use of the chest to limit the "downstroke" of the diaphragm, as Lamaze put it, claiming that pregnant women feel pain on deep inspiration. Yet proponents of shallow breathing who believe that the diaphragm irritates the uterus during the first stage of labor also believe that it acts as a piston to push out the baby in the second stage of labor! How strange that internal structures, peaceful neighbors all along, suddenly conflict during labor. Mammals have a diaphragm precisely so that breathing, which occurs in the chest, can continue during activity of the abdominal and other muscles.

Tense, anxious people breathe with their chests and shoulders, instead of with their diaphragms, which is the more physiological way. Likewise, chest breathing leads to feelings of anxiety and tension, which interferes with an expectant mother's ability to relax and remain aware of her feelings. Rapid and shallow breathing, through over-oxygenation and increased muscular activity, diminishes body awareness. The repetition of such breathing patterns during labor, a time of stress, requires continual effort. (You can check for yourself how this effort interferes with relaxation by altering your breathing rhythm for a few minutes.) Furthermore, two specific problems develop as a result of artificial breathing. These are hypoventilation (underbreathing) and hyperventilation (overbreathing). While brief periods of one or the other may not be harmful, the cumulative effects on both mother and child need to be considered, especially if there are other interferences in the labor (such as medication, anesthesia, backlying position).

Anxiety is the experience of breathing difficulty during any blocked excitement.
FREDERICK PERLS

Tonic contraction of the diaphragm is expressed in individuals with shallow and interrupted breathing.
KEN DYCHTWALD

Hypoventilation

Underbreathing occurs when respiration is kept very shallow, such as with light, quick panting recommended by educators for active labor. There is inadequate oxygen intake and carbon dioxide, the major regulator of respiration, is washed out, which means there is less stimulus for oxygen intake. Breathing, especially during labor, must be deep enough so that sufficient air can traverse the anatomical dead space for gaseous exchange in the lungs. The anatomical dead space extends from the nostrils through the windpipe and branches of the bronchi to the air sacs, which are the outposts of lung tissue.

Hyperventilation

Overbreathing results in surplus oxygen being circulated in the body. This disturbance of physiology occurs when excessive oxygen is inhaled (during "cleansing" breaths,* or with the use of an oxygen mask). Hyperventilation also occurs if there is normal oxygen intake, but carbon dioxide levels are lowered (such as during forceful blowing in labor, or inflating an air mattress). Carbon dioxide, a waste product, widens blood vessels to facilitate its own removal. During hyperventilation, there is a decrease in the relative amount of carbon dioxide, and blood vessels therefore become constricted. The surplus oxygen causes the blood to become more alkaline, impairing the release of oxygen from the hemoglobin in the red blood cells that transports it.

The paradoxical result of hyperventilation is that although the mother is taking in surplus oxygen, the combination of these two effects means less blood flow carrying less oxygen to the tissues. If circulation to the uterus and placenta is decreased, then the baby can suffer from a lack of oxygen. This situation is more likely if there is a fall in maternal cardiac output from other causes, such as backlying or epidural anesthesia. Clinical symptoms associated with hyperventilation include slowing of the fetal heart and a build-up of waste products, causing fetal circulation to be more acid. Fetal distress leads to intervention in labor, often caesarean delivery.

Typically, hyperventilation occurs with rapid, deep breathing that accelerates at the peak of a contraction's intensity. Accelerated breathing patterns sound like a train

---

* The "cleansing" breath is typically performed at the start and end of each contraction as a way to sign on and off. British childbirth educator and author Sheila Kitzinger makes a good point when she asks, "What is it we are supposed to be cleansing?"

passing, as the breath follows the waxing and waning of the contraction. Of course, it is normal for respiration to adapt to any physical exertion, whether in labor or jogging. If women are taught to accelerate their breathing in prenatal classes, then they will do so even more during the actual labor. At rest, the frequency of normal breathing ranges from about five to twenty-two breaths per minute. Researchers at the Bristol Maternity Hospital in England found that mothers trained in psychoprophylactic breathing patterns took over one hundred breaths per minute during labor!

Deep inhalation increases reflex activity and dams up biological energy in the vegetative centers.
WILHELM REICH

Emphasis on inhalation, such as the "cleansing" breath, can disturb the balance of blood gases. Preferably, the outward breath is emphasized. Exhalation is the natural relaxation phase of the respiratory cycle and no one can exhale too much air. The next inhaled breath is physiologically regulated to replace the amount of exhaled air.

The body of a laboring woman has the wisdom to regulate itself by breaking through breath-control techniques. During pregnancy, the threshold of the respiratory center in the brain is lowered. Women are more susceptible to blood gas disturbances, medication, and anesthesia at this time. Frequently, in prenatal class, and in labor, women complain that they feel "all out of air" or that they "have to stop and take in a deep breath," which is the normal reaction to an oxygen debt. The body's last resort against hyperventilation is fainting. This enables the involuntary centers of respiration to reestablish equilibrium while the mind is temporarily out of action. Most of us are aware of symptoms that result from diminished blood flow after hyperventilation. Side effects include visual clouding, dizziness, tingling in the fingers or lips, even muscle spasms in the hands and feet.

Many mothers do not give themselves credit for coping with labor and swear by the success of breathing patterns. Invariably, these are the very women whose labors were not long or difficult. Unphysiological breathing may not matter much in a brief, easy labor, but it becomes depleting if labor is prolonged. In most cases a laboring mother needs to conserve the flow of her energy. Women who have prolonged, hard labors cannot sustain exaggerated respiratory patterns.

Breath-Holding

To hold one's breath is to hold oneself back. People with good body mechanics or intuitive physical awareness do not hold their breath during exercise or physical exertion. A baby manages all kinds of feats without interrupting his or her breathing, or tensing unnecessary muscles. Children, as they grow up, commonly develop the habit of fixing the diaphragm to control their emotions and "gut" feelings, by holding their breath and tightening their abdominal walls.

Every disturbance of the ability to fully experience one's own body damages self-confidence, as well as the unity of bodily feeling. At the same time, it creates the need for compensation.
WILHELM REICH

Children also learn breath-holding and the use of accessory muscles when premature toilet training is enforced. Breath-holding thus becomes associated with tension, discomfort, and an inability to let go. While elimination should involve only the physical act of letting something pass from the body, habits of strain and effort easily become deeply entrenched. Children on toilets strain to please their parents. Women in labor are made to strain to please their obstetricians. Even without the desired result from a child or woman in labor, the obvious effort reassures parents and birth attendants and encourages their praise.

Respiratory inhibition that begins in childhood continues in adults who have trouble accepting the body's sexual and excretory functions. It is also a way to suppress deep feelings. Most of us have grown up forcing ourselves to compensate for movements that no longer happen naturally. We are so accustomed to control that the idea of spontaneity is often frightening. It is no surprise, then, that expectant couples latch on to the ideas of control and effort for childbirth preparation to avoid their coming to terms with their intense emotions, fears, and the unpredictable nature of birth.

Patients have concocted every conceivable means of preventing deep exhalation.
WILHELM REICH

Buried emotions easily surface with the ability to permit (not force) a complete exhalation — a total letting go of the breath, the body, and the self. Many forms of therapy,

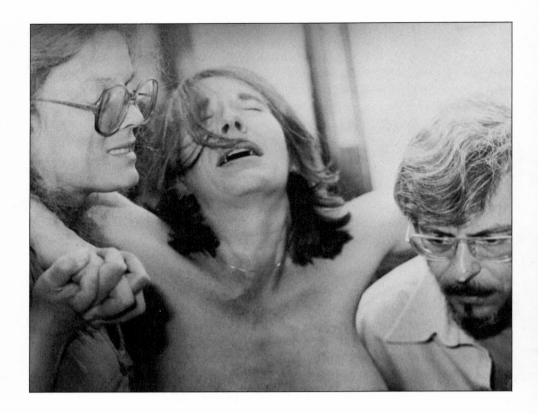

such as Bioenergetics, Rebirthing, and Primal Therapy, actually emphasize freeing the breath, to resolve tension and energy blocks. Similarly, a turning point occurs during an exercise program when the individual notices that his or her breath flows freely with any movement and does not have to be consciously released anymore. Most adults hold their breath while exercising because they feel this is the way to do their best and to exert themselves fully. A great many people even believe that exercise is only beneficial if it hurts. On the contrary, the deeper rewards of exercise come from achieving less and experiencing more. Pain is a warning signal. Breath-holding during physical exertion can be dangerous, such as during diving, particularly if the diving follows a period of hyperventilation. Weightlifters and practitioners of the martial arts, for example, learn the importance of the exhaled breath. The weightlifter who grunts during a final hoist is using his abdominal muscles to brace and protect his spine, as these muscles can only shorten on outward breath. In karate, the force of the blow is also developed on a vocalized exhalation. In T'ai Chi, there is an elastic strength that emerges through a flowing, yielding use of breath and body.

It seems odd that physiological principles well understood in sport and exercise are actually reversed in obstetrics. The conventional "management" of the second stage of labor, when the uterine contractions expel the baby down the vaginal canal, makes no sense at all. The mother is made to hold her breath, fix her chest, tense her shoulders, stiffen her neck, and concentrate her effort on command. Although many people are used to the daily ritual of forcing their bowels, others find straining uncomfortable and self-defeating. (Imagine, as you are reading this, how you would react if told you had to move your bowels within the next five minutes.)

Downward fixation of the diaphragm and tension of the abdominal wall blocks biological energy . . . suppresses pleasurable sensations as well as curtailing abdominal anxiety.
WILHELM REICH

Labor is one time when the cues from the body are immediate and powerful. Why isn't support for a laboring woman simple encouragement and patience for her to do what she feels is natural? Perhaps one reason is because the sounds that a laboring woman makes may be the same as she makes approaching orgasm.* A display of sexuality is not considered appropriate in a clinical setting, where shaving of the mother's pubic hair, draping her body, and restraint of her vocalizations, movements, and partner contact have been routine procedures changing only slowly. Instead, tension and breath-holding, together with a tight pelvic floor typically seen in second-stage labor, are common to the bodily pattern of sexual repression. Wilhelm Reich noticed that sexually inhibited persons hold their breath and either keep their bodies still or make forced movements, hollowing the back forward to withdraw the genital area. Birthing women sometimes do this

True freedom means no internal choice — the seed contains within it its own demand for action.
JOEL KRAMER

Sexuality and anxiety are functions of living organisms operating in opposite directions; pleasurable expansion and anxious contraction.
WILHELM REICH

* When Dr. Frederick Leboyer first showed his film *Birth Without Violence* in Boston, many people in the audience were unsettled by the moans of the birthing woman and commented that she seemed to be in pain. After some time, one brave viewer suggested, to Leboyer's obvious relief and appreciation, that the mother's vocalizations were just like the spontaneous sounds of lovemaking.

by arching their backs, as a result of being made to hold their bodies rigid and to force their pushing.

BREATH-HOLDING IN THE SECOND STAGE OF LABOR

Reflexes do not manifest themselves properly when voluntary skeletal muscles are involved unless conscious control is smoothly and completely withdrawn.
MOSHE FELDENKRAIS

During birth, women are usually made to push harder and longer than is necessary and are often told to do so before their natural pushing urges have developed. Frequently, the less a mother's desire to push, the more the staff encourage her to strain. The baby's head is usually still high in the pelvis at this point, particularly if it is a first baby. Only when the baby's head has descended low enough to stimulate the stretch receptors in the pelvic floor muscles does the mother feel the urge to push. The pushing may take some time to become established (allowing the mother a peaceful interlude) and it is wise for her to conserve her energy until her sensation to push becomes irresistible.

Most obstetricians are concerned about their tight schedules and statistical guidelines for the length of second-stage labor. Therefore, they generally insist on forced pushing and may even threaten to use forceps. Well-meaning nurses know that the doctors will in fact intervene if the labor does not progress according to the obstetrician's standard, so nurses often encourage the mother to strain as hard as she can. Childbirth educators, knowing these hospital practices, generally advise couples in class to push when the doctor or nurse commands, even though in pregnancy they may have warned against rehearsals of pushing with the breath held.

The majority of childbirth educators are coming to appreciate that forced pushing with breath-holding is undesirable. While some mothers need to work hard to get a large baby's head through their pelvises or to rotate a baby whose head is in a difficult position, they do not need to hold their breath. The abdominal muscles, in fact, work best on outward breath.

Laboring women are often rolled into a flexed position on their backs. Energy is wasted during birth because a mother's legs have to be held up by her arms. Pulling on the legs tenses the whole body, as anyone can feel by assuming this unnatural position. In addition, if the mother is flat on her back, she has to push the baby uphill through her pelvis, against the force of gravity. Although backlying remains a common birth position, progressive doctors and midwives now encourage women to assume more functional, upright positions such as squatting or kneeling.

Breath-Holding and Straining Disturbs Physiology

When respiration is interrupted there is no oxygenation. Straining with the breath held produces marked cardiovascular effects. This forced effort with a closed glottis is known as the Valsalva maneuver, named after a seventeenth-century Italian physician who recommended the technique for expelling pus from the middle ear. Old people have died straining on bedpans, and there have been rare reports of strokes and even death in laboring women who were made to strain excessively during birth. A few moments of strain, though giving no advantage to the laboring woman, is usually not harmful. However, if the Valsalva maneuver is prolonged beyond about six seconds, then maternal and fetal physiology are affected. Disturbances include less blood flow to the placenta, slowing of the fetal heart rate, and an increased chance of caesarean delivery due to fetal distress. (See Appendix 1, page 121.)

Blocking the breath during any exertion produces a closed pressure system like a balloon. The key factor is the breath-holding. If air is released, however slowly (such as with a grunt or a groan), then the Valsalva maneuver is avoided. The difference is subtle but significant. However, labor attendants are usually alarmed if they hear any sounds from the woman while she pushes. Noise indicates to them that air is escaping and the mother's pushing force is waning.

Determined and fruitless bearing-down diminishes the elasticity of the pelvic tissues.
GRANTLY DICK-READ

During the Valsalva maneuver, very high pressures created in the chest prevent the blood in the large veins of the pelvis and abdomen from returning to the heart. Therefore, there is less blood to circulate to the mother's lungs, the rest of her body, and the placenta. Her blood pressure, which was very high at the onset of strain, falls as a result. When breakpoint is reached, various protective mechanisms are aroused and the poor victim gasps with relief. Until the cardiovascular system returns to normal, there is an overshoot phenomenon, which causes imbalance of pressure throughout the various body fluids. Abnormal changes in brain waves and heart rates have been recorded on research subjects, usually young, healthy men performing handgrip tests for just a few seconds. This requires much less exertion than is required by laboring women as they lie, usually on their backs, trying to give birth.

When the Valsalva maneuver is used, it is common to see a mother with a purple face, bloodshot eyes, and burst capillaries in her cheeks. The labor staff and coach assemble like a cheering squad, and with the kindest of intentions, exhort the mother to *push! push! push! push!* At the same time, they command this flexed ball of tension to relax. Readers need only to get down on the floor and try relaxing while straining with the breath held to realize how impossible this combination is.

If you hold your breath and strain, you will feel the muscles of your pelvic floor protectively tighten in response to the pressure from above. This has also been shown by direct muscle research. Dr. Roberto Caldeyro-Barcia recently investigated the effects of pushing. He found that bearing-down efforts are always longer and more forceful when the mother is made to push than if she responds spontaneously to the contractions. Forced pushing is also associated with the need for an episiotomy. If there is insufficient time and relaxation, then the perineum is not able to distend adequately. The center seam of the abdominal wall, where the recti muscles* unite (and sometimes separate) is also strained. Other complications following a forceful second-stage labor include pelvic floor dysfunction, with prolapse of the bladder, bowel, or uterus. The mechanism by which this occurs was pointed out in 1957 by a British obstetrician, Dr. Constance Bey-

---

* See *Essential Exercises for the Childbearing Year*, Second ed., Revised, for a discussion of the rectus abdominus muscles.

non. She uses the analogy of the lining in a coat sleeve being dragged down, to describe how pelvic structural supports are weakened when forced downward from pressure above.

A considerable amount of blood pools in the pelvis during the Valsalva maneuver, because the blood cannot return to the heart against the high pressure in the chest. The veins, which in pregnancy are dilated more easily due to hormonal softening, are thus predisposed to varicosities such as hemorrhoids.

If the strain is prolonged (and women in labor are usually told to hold their breath for at least twenty seconds), low blood pressure results. If a series of Valsalva maneuvers are demanded, then the blood pressure is raised. Fortunately, women in labor rarely hold their breath for as long as they are taught or told to do.

Conducted in such a manner, the second stage of labor has been limited to one and a half to two hours, with good reason. Could mother and baby stand much of this stress and strain? Dr. Vellay wrote that "the mother brings the baby into the world instead of waiting for it to come by itself." Today, holistic doctors and midwives feel that birth has its own rhythms, which should be respected, and enough time and appropriate timing for the mother's pushes must be allowed.

Birthing the baby's head may receive little emphasis in childbirth classes, because by late-second-stage labor the doctor is present and conducting the delivery. In most cases, a mother is instructed to pant while an episiotomy is cut and her baby is born. Episiotomy has become almost routine in modern obstetric practice. However, in the Netherlands and in the U.S.A., with supportive attendants who permit the mother to give birth in her own style, episiotomies or tears are the exception rather than the rule.

Episiotomy, deservedly known as the "unkind cut," is a controversial surgical procedure that in itself is the subject of whole books. Women should know that there are no controlled studies showing any benefits from this vaginal incision, which may extend to the anus. Episiotomy is the major cause of blood loss and infection at birth. Proper, careful suturing of the perineum takes a long time and interferes with the postpartum bonding of the new family. Poor anatomical repair is common and the pain from this incision, usually done without a mother's informed consent, may persist for weeks or months, contributing to sexual problems and postpartum depression. Painkillers, which affect the breast milk, are routinely prescribed. The impact of this genital mutilation on a woman's self-image and sexuality can be severe. Everything from sitting to bowel movements to lovemaking is painful and difficult for her.

While there are a small percentage of cases in which an episiotomy may be required (such as when the baby is in distress), there is no justification for the present near-universal rate of this surgery. Dr. David Banta of the Office of Technology Assessment of the United States Congress reviewed more than 250 articles on the subject of episiotomy and concluded that the risks outweighed the benefits.

Many skilled midwives believe that perineal tears are less traumatic, less extensive, and heal better than the physician's "neat cut." Muscles tear along lines of least resistance and heal better than incisions as any woman who has experienced both can testify. Minor tears do not require stitches at all. Another misconception is that episiotomy prevents future pelvic-floor problems. This is not confirmed by any scientific evidence. In older generations and in countries where the episiotomy rate is low, such as the Netherlands, there is less, not more, reconstructive surgery for pelvic-floor dysfunction. Second, the incidence of pelvic-floor problems and surgery in the United States has not dropped since episiotomy became routine.

Time for Change

The nature of labor and delivery for each expectant couple remains unknown until it happens. Although the introduction of labor-management techniques was based on a sincere assumption of the value and necessity of a mother's mental control over the physical experience of birth, the techniques are now controversial or outdated. Good intentions easily become interventions. Many people today seek education and therapy to get in touch with their bodies, to free their anxiety and breathing, to simplify their existence, and to become more aware of their inner feelings. It seems paradoxical that expectant couples, at this very expansive and sentient time of their lives, are learning to hold themselves back instead of opening up to go with the flow.

The gift of insight — of making imaginative new connections — once the specialty of a lucky few, is there for anyone willing to persist, experiment and explore.
MARILYN FERGUSON

The childbearing year is a time of tremendous personal growth. Childbirth educators who appreciate the psycho-physiological dimensions of pregnancy and birth can act as catalysts so that growth can flourish. Techniques that develop a couple's awareness of the here and now and their unspoken fears are a world apart from training in techniques to be used during the labor, an event in the future. Childbirth education, with regard to a program for the birth experience, can be likened to a menu. When you go to a restaurant you have no control over the kitchen and no idea how the food is until it arrives on your plate. Similarly, recipes for birth often don't turn out the way one expects.

She learns her task as she goes along.
GRANTLY DICK-READ

Childbirth preparation that takes preparation for the unexpected into account makes it easier for pregnant parents to accept their individual labors and confront the unknown. Instead of spending time in class practicing one-time techniques of questionable value, they can explore the full range of experience offered by pregnancy and birth and learn how to assert their wishes in a hospital environment.

Resources

Books and Articles

HOSPITAL INTERVENTIONS

Bean, Constance. *Labor and Delivery: An Observer's Diary: What You Should Know About Today's Childbirth.* Garden City, N.Y.: Doubleday, 1977. Factual accounts about what happens in hospitals. Also discusses homebirth and circumcision.

Haire, Doris. *The Cultural Warping of Childbirth.* A special report by International Childbirth Education Association, 1972. Available from ICEA, P.O. Box 20048, Minneapolis, MN 55426. Documented criticism of many routine obstetric procedures; shows how poorly the U.S. measures up to other countries.

Kitzinger, Sheila, ed. *Episiotomy — Physical and Emotional Aspects.* London: National Childbirth Trust, 9 Queensborough Terr., London W2, England, 1981. (Available from ICEA, P.O. Box 20048, Minneapolis, MN 55426.) Articles by different professionals on the use and misuse of episiotomy and its many undesirable side effects.

UNDERSTANDING THE BODY

Benson, Herbert, M.D. *The Mind-Body Effect.* New York: Berkeley, 1981. A clear explanation of how the body's mental and physical processes interact.

————. *The Relaxation Response.* New York: Berkeley, 1978. Simple description of how meditation techniques benefit the body.

Caldeyro-Barcia, Roberto, M.D. "The Influence of Maternal Position on Labor" and "The Influence of Maternal Bearing-Down Efforts in the Second Stage of Labor on Fetal Well-Being," in *Kaleidoscope of Childbearing: Preparation, Birth and Nurturing,* eds. Simkin, Penny, and Carla Reinke. Seattle: the pennypress, 1978. Scientific documentation of the benefits of upright positions and spontaneous pushing without breath-holding in childbirth.

Huxley, Aldous. *The Art of Seeing.* Seattle: Montana Books, 1975. A holistic view of vision and its interaction with breathing, posture, and relaxation.

Morgan, William. "The Mind of the Marathoners," *Psychology Today,* April 1978. How marathon winners learn to associate instead of dissociating from their pain in running.

Noble, Elizabeth. "Controversies in Maternal Effort During Labor and Delivery," *Journal of Nurse-Midwifery* 26:2 (March/April 1981). Evaluation of maternal position, controlled breathing, and forced pushing in second stage, and suggested alternatives.

————. "Respiratory Considerations for Childbirth," in *Kaleidoscope of Childbearing: Preparation, Birth and Nurturing,* eds. Simkin, Penny, and Carla Reinke. Seattle: the pennypress, 1978. Physiological effects of hyperventilation and the Valsalva maneuver.

CHAPTER 4

The Natural Flow of Labor and Birth

BIRTH IS always the same, yet it is always different. Like a sunset, the mystery is also the appeal to those who get up in the middle of the night to attend laboring women. While the sequence of birth is simple, the nature of the experience is complex and unique to each individual. No matter how much any of us may know about births in general, we know nothing about a particular labor and delivery until it occurs.

The entire birth process is normally achieved by involuntary muscular contractions. The muscles of the uterus dilate the cervix, creating an entry to the vagina. When the opening is wide enough to permit the baby's head to pass through, the uterus pushes the baby down through the birth canal. The fetal head turns and the skull bones are squeezed so that the head can fit through the different contours of the pelvis. The final stage of labor is completed with the arrival of the afterbirth, the placenta and membranes.

Three stages of labor have been identified in modern obstetrics for the purpose of clinical management. Even substages have been categorized, such as prodromal labor (warning signs), active phase, and accelerated labor, when the uterus is really moving along toward full dilation. Nature, however, is not controlled by the way it is studied. Labor, like pregnancy, is a process and does not start and

I like to use the term "rush" in place of "contraction" because I think it describes better how to flow with the birthing energy.
INA MAY GASKIN

stop with systems of measurement. The clinical usefulness of the conventional definitions of the stages of labor needs reevaluation.

Second stage is said to begin when the cervix is fully dilated. Complete dilation is defined as ten centimeters, or five fingers, in diameter. This assessment is made by vaginal examination. When the cervix is felt to be fully open, the mother is typically exhorted to push her baby out as hard and as fast as possible, certainly within two hours. If we consider second stage to begin when the mother feels a natural urge to push, it would change the whole management of labor. In the *Barefoot Doctor's Manual* the Chinese describe only two divisions of labor. One ends with the birth of the baby and the other ends with the delivery of the placenta. Midwives have traditionally done very few internal examinations to assess the progress of labor. Instead, they see labor as a process and rely on their intuition and observation of the woman.

Childbirth educators have their own evaluations of the stages of labor, such as "transition is the toughest time" or "second stage is usually the short, easy part." In fact, the term *transition,* which is not found in any obstetric text, can become a self-fulfilling prophecy. The mother almost looks forward to feeling nausea, shivering, sweating, trembling, irritation, and other symptoms attributed to the end of first stage, because then she believes the worst is over.

While the sequence of events in labor is the same, the nature of them is extremely varied. Labor can be long, slow, easy, hard, pleasurable, painful, lonely, or joyous. Membranes can rupture early or late; babies can arrive at all times. A small number of women give birth hastily and perhaps unattended. The most open-minded educators and couples, then, accept the fact that despite the best planning, labor is an individual experience and is always a journey into the unknown.

An important point for expectant couples to keep in mind about birth is not so much what may happen in labor, but what should be avoided so that the natural process may unfold without interference. Because birth is a unique process it is easier to define what is undesirable rather than what is desirable.

Medication and Anesthesia

Drug usage is easily rationalized by the medical view of pregnancy, an illness best managed by specialist physicians in a hospital. However, in the absence of birth complications, it is essential for a mother to avoid taking any drugs. Medication and anesthesia produce side effects that can play havoc with the checks and balances of normal birth. They depress the central nervous system, making the mother less aware. Regional anesthesia, such as an epidural, can cause fetal distress through a fall in the mother's blood pressure. In general, the progress of labor slows down, making the labor longer and more difficult. Instruments may be needed for delivery as a result.

If all the drugs in Pharmacopia, with a few exceptions, were thrown into the sea, it would be better for mankind and worse for the fishes.
OLIVER WENDELL HOLMES

Drugs lead to more drugs. A painkilling drug may diminish contractions, so a stimulant is given to augment them. Next, the labor may become very intense, requiring more painkillers. A vicious circle ensues. In addition to the adverse effect on labor, all drugs cross the placenta and we may never know all the effects they can have on a baby's developing brain.

Laboring women are tempted to take drugs, which are often pressed on them, because of their fear and pain. It is more expedient for busy nurses to administer a few shots of medication than to provide comfort and support, which also make pain bearable. Drugs and anesthesia render a laboring woman passive and motionless to enable the doctor to *deliver* the baby. If mothers knew the side effects of these drugs, the great majority would refuse them. There is no medication that is both safe and effective. Most drugs used in labor have not been adequately tested because using pregnant women as subjects is contrary to medical ethics. Physicians' use of the same untested drugs in pregnancy and birth apparently is acceptable!

The Committee on Drugs of the American Academy of Pediatrics has cautioned that there is no drug, whether an over-the-counter remedy or a prescription drug, which, when taken by or administered to a pregnant woman, has been proved to be without risk to the unborn infant.
DORIS HAIRE

The physical experience of birth, like that of pregnancy,

is crucial to mother-infant bonding and a woman's transition to motherhood. Thousands of women who were drugged and anesthetized for this rite of passage have expressed long-lasting regrets over the effects on their family relationships as well as on their own emotional well-being. The mind may know that a baby was born, but the body and heart feel cheated. As mothers often comment after a spinal or epidural, "It's like watching a birth on TV."

The Environment of Birth

Choosing the place of and attendants for birth should be a personal and well-considered decision. Options vary in different communities and include home, birth centers, hospital birthing rooms, midwives, family practitioners, obstetricians, and the presence of friends, relatives, and other children. The traditional hospital arrangement is the least desirable, for the drama of birth is played out there in five different places. Women are admitted in one area, labor in another, deliver in a third, recover in a fourth, and then are moved to the postpartum floor. Studies of laboring mice and ewes showed that movement or disturbance causes prolonged labor and higher death rates in their offspring. We may speculate that human beings are perhaps even more sensitive, rather than less so.

A suitable birth environment is one that is quiet, calm, warm, and comfortable. The smells, sounds, and colors of a place for the sick are reassuring only to those women who feel secure when surrounded by uniformed professionals and high-tech medical equipment. More progressive birth rooms have double beds for the comfort and intimacy of the couple. Some are like a small apartment, with an attached bathroom and kitchenette, so that a family can live together during the mother's stay. Other couples may remain in the birth environment for just a few hours before returning home.

Labor Support

First-time expectant parents prepare for birth today as if going into battle. One battle is with the mother's body. Another battle is with the hospital staff and policies if the couple's needs are not met or if they have to ward off obstetrical interference. The less homelike the environment, and the more rules the institution imposes, the more a couple need to know their rights and options beforehand.

A 1980 study published in the *New England Journal of Medicine* noted the positive effects of a supportive labor companion and suggested there may be an association between acute maternal anxiety and arrests of labor or fetal distress. Fear, stress, and negative emotions can depress uterine activity through the action of chemicals secreted by the body, called catecholamines, and adrenalin, which works against the body's uterine stimulant, oxytocin.

Women can "un-dilate" with one unkind glance.
INA MAY GASKIN

A support person who accompanies the parents can act as an advocate for them during labor. The mother and her partner are not in a strong position to assert themselves against medical intervention as they are absorbed in the physical and emotional experiences of birthing. A great many couples feel afraid and inferior when surrounded by professional authorities. Documenting their wishes in the form of a birth plan kept with the mother's chart is a good way to have issues squared away in advance and written down to prevent conflict. (See Appendix 7, page 132.) Perhaps mothers could also make their wishes clear to hospital staff by wearing a series of buttons on their labor gowns stating NO EPIDURAL, NO FETAL MONITOR, and the like!

Birthing with insight, a mother freely finds her own labor positions, makes sounds without inhibition, enjoys support and caresses from her partner and chosen attendants, eats to appetite, drinks to thirst, and generally responds in a way that feels natural for her. In a liberal birth environment, such as an alternative birth center or at home, she does not have to worry about how her behavior is viewed by others or whether she is conforming to a certain method of birth.

The art of helping a woman in labor is no mystery. A support person merely need listen to his or her common sense and nurturing instincts. After all, if an exhausted hiker landed on the doorstep, most people would know how to offer physical assistance, warmth, nourishment, rest, and moral support. Yet labor is often an isolated, lonely experience with most of a woman's bodily and emotional needs totally ignored. Women easily become dehydrated with the work of labor and require fluids. Various types of fruit juice or noncaffeine teas are more refreshing and palatable than an intravenous drip. Easily digested foods such as mashed potatoes, soups with rice, or the type of high-carbohydrate liquid snack that marathon runners take en route all help to keep up a mother's energy levels during labor.*

Comfort measures that may be available in the home need some promotion in the hospital environment. These include beanbag chairs that can be easily shaped for body support and a large mattress or futon so that the mother's body can be comfortable massaged by one or more persons if she desires. As well as aiding relaxation, massage raises the pain threshold. According to the "gate control" theory of pain, stimulation of nerve pathways in the skin cause faster impulses to crowd the "control gate" in the nervous system before the slower pain messages arrive.

Plenty of pillows are needed during labor, with some to be used in the bath for long soaks. Hospitals, alas, generally offer access only to a shower. Dr. Michel Odent, in his clinic in Pithiviers, France, encourages laboring women to relax in a warm pool. Frequently, the mothers refuse to come out and there have been dozens of unplanned underwater births. Dr. Odent always lifts the baby to the surface immediately to establish breathing. No problems have resulted from the underwater birthings.

---

* Food has traditionally been withheld from laboring women in hospitals because of the potential hazard that the stomach contents could be inhaled under general anesthesia. However, the great majority of caesareans are done with regional anesthesia (spinal or epidural), and in the rare cases when a general anesthetic is required, a tube is put down the mother's throat to prevent aspiration of vomit. It is widely thought that digestion stops during labor, but the research on which that opinion is based was done on laboring mothers who had received medication.

Planned underwater homebirths are starting to receive publicity in the United States. Usually both parents are together in a hot tub of distilled water, to which some salt has been added to approximate amniotic fluid. Often the baby is allowed to take its time to move around in the water after birth. As long as the placenta has not separated, oxygen is supplied to the baby through the pulsing umbilical cord. (The cord ceases to pulsate much sooner when in contact with air, as the jelly inside the cord then hardens to clamp off the blood vessels.) Parents may well debate what the exact time of such a birth is!

A rocking chair, a high stool for the mother to lean on, and a hard-backed chair for counterpressure during contractions may come in handy during labor. A horseshoe-shaped stool, used for yoga headstands, makes an appropriate support for the pushing phase of labor because of the open front. A lounge chair for squatting is another option. Arm supports are available and between pushes the mother can sit up on the top of the chair back to rest. Soft lighting, candles, music, even incense, are used during labor to aid relaxation, depending, of course, on the mother's wishes.

Some couples want birth to be shared with friends and relatives; others want a private and intimate experience. Sensitivity to the emotional and sexual needs of the expectant parents and basic good manners, such as knocking on doors, are essential from labor attendants. While people can bring energy to a birth, they can also draw energy away from the mother. The ability of the birth attendants to resonate with the mother's needs and feelings is an important, although intangible, quality. Persons offering labor support have to *be* there for the mother, spiritually as well as physically, but they may be caught up with unresolved feelings about their own births.

Favorable Positions for Labor and Birth

Standing and walking in labor are preferred by the majority of women, although in childbirth classes most labor rehearsals take place with couples lying on the floor. Hospitals are now starting to permit women to get out of bed and move around because of the overwhelming evidence that upright positions assist the progress of labor. Of course, it is difficult for a woman to be mobile if she is attached to an electronic fetal monitor or an intravenous drip.

When a laboring woman lies flat on her back, her uterus compresses major blood vessels (increased by contractions) and the circulation to the heart is impaired. This causes a drop in her blood pressure. As a result, the blood flow to the uterus and placenta diminishes so that fetal distress — a drop in the baby's heart rate — is likely. Respiration is also hampered when a laboring woman lies on her back, which psychologically is a claustrophobic and vulnerable position.

Research has proved that walking shortens labor and lessens the need for drugs to relieve pain or stimulate contractions. Walking causes fewer abnormalities of the fetal heart rate and less molding of the fetal skull bones, which are compressed during the birth process.

If the mother prefers to sit or lie on her side, she should be encouraged to do so — she must be guided by her comfort and what feels right for her body. Some women need to rest in labor, others want to be more active. All mothers must have the option to move around freely during labor and delivery.

Dr. Caldeyro-Barcia has studied the influence of maternal position on labor. He found that labors were 25 percent shorter and the mothers experienced less pain when they were allowed simply to recline with their bodies at an angle of about 40 degrees, instead of lying horizontal. Furthermore, gravity had the added effect of increasing the efficiency of the contractions. (See Appendix 2, page 122.)

The drive angle of the uterus is important in the mechanics of labor. The axis of the fetal spine, together with the axis of the maternal spine, form an angle between 60 and 80 degrees in the upright position. The uterus tips slightly forward during contractions and the drive angle in an upright position helps to direct the fetal head toward the back of the pelvis. If the mother is lying flat on her back, this angle is decreased. The weaker contractions direct the fetal head toward the front of the pelvis, which may lead to delay and difficulties with the labor. (See Appendix 3, page 123.)

The recent revival of birth chairs is a welcome improvement over the labor bed and flat delivery table, although substituting one piece of equipment for another, however superior, does not offer women all the birth options they may seek. Furthermore, if the mother rests on any part of her pelvis or her perineum, as in a sitting or half-lying position, there is a counterforce acting against the descent of her baby. Dr. Michel Odent offers his clients a room devoid of any furniture except a platform and pillows so that no birth positions are suggested. He prefers to encourage a mother to listen to her body and assume the position that seems appropriate for her. In the United States, birth chairs cost thousands of dollars, but in Sao Paulo, Brazil, Dr. Celia De Vale uses a chair that was specially built at a cost of less than one hundred dollars.

Squatting, kneeling, standing, hanging supported from the arms, all fours, and side-lying are some positions women choose for labor and birth, in addition to the traditional reclining posture. For over one hundred years, anthropologists have documented that while there is no universal position for birth, free choice of backlying is conspicuous by its absence.

Squatting, while uncomfortable for most people without prior practice, offers one of the most functional positions for birth. According to studies in Sweden by Dr. Christian Ehrstrom, when a mother squats the pelvic outlet is at its widest, increased by one to two centimeters. The pelvis is completely tilted to align with the spine, making the most curved passage for the baby's descent. The contraction of the abdominal muscles is very efficient in squatting as they are in a shortened, middle position of their range. Not only does gravity provide additional force from above, but there is no counterforce from below. The vagina becomes shorter and wider, and less effort is required by the mother to open up and let the baby out at her own pace. During crowning of the baby's head, there is an equal stretch all around the perineum, so that this muscular membranous "cuff" is least likely to tear or to require enlargement by an episiotomy. Women who squat for birth can generally deliver their babies without any manual assistance at all. Gravity and the free space around the perineum allow the baby's rotation maneuvers to be accomplished spontaneously.

Squatting and the all fours position are the safest and easiest ways to deliver a breech (where the baby presents with the lower part of the body instead of the head).

An excellent film (listed in the Resources, page 92) made in a modern Brazilian hospital shows several unassisted deliveries in the squatting position. Such visual education generates self-confidence in women, as they see they *can* give birth by themselves. This brief but remarkable film conveys the essence of birth. It stands out in contrast to the standard prepared childbirth movies that present the roles of the team members and all the props of birth that enable the doctor to get the baby out.

Dr. Odent noted that women often adopt an asymmetrical position for labor. This makes sense because, until just before the birth, the baby's head is always to the left or to the right side of the mother's pelvis. Rocking and rolling movements also help the mother to work with the contraction to facilitate the descent and rotation of the baby's head. As one physician commented, "You don't pull out a cork, or take off a ring, without twisting and turning," and a baby's head fits very snugly in the pelvis.

The Momentum of Labor

The uterus does not only contract in labor. It contracts during menstruation, orgasm, pregnancy (Braxton-Hicks contractions), labor, and postpartum, when it is returning to its normal size. ("After-pains" are felt more with second and subsequent births, supposedly because the uterus has been stretched more often and therefore has to contract very strongly to return to its original size.)

Established and progressive contractions form the cardinal sign of labor. It is not exactly understood how labor is triggered, although it can be artificially induced with the drug pitocin (synthetic oxytocin) or prostaglandins. Some researchers believe that fetal hormones also contribute to the onset of labor. Loss of the mucus plug ("bloody show") that seals off the cervix and leakage of the amniotic fluid surrounding the baby are signs that labor is imminent. However, actual contractions may not follow for hours or days. Contractions are the muscular work of the uterus, which will birth the baby. They occur in waves, with rest intervals between them, which makes pain more bearable. Like a symphony, there are various moods and movements in labor, but in true labor there is a pattern of increasing intensity, with contractions growing longer, stronger, and closer together, later opening the cervix and expelling the baby.

The uterus works involuntarily, but it is very sensitive to discord in the mother's body and mind. Labors can slow down and even stop in reaction to such things as a change in the external environment during admission to hospital or negative attitudes in outsiders, family, friends, or the mother herself. Sometimes she may have flashbacks to her own birth, which can affect how she responds to her own labor. Labors can be speeded up — for example, when the membranes rupture or by a birth attendant's vaginal examination. It also helps if the mother stands or walks around, takes a hot shower, has a massage, or a good cry.

The mother's psychological experience of this physical process is as variable as the course of labor itself. Primarily, it depends on how she has come to terms with her fear and anxiety during pregnancy and how she views the sexuality of birth. Whether she sees her labor as interminably long and agonizing or slow but progressing normally, for example, relates to her state of mind. A skillful birth attendant or close friend can encourage the mother to work through deep feelings that hold back the labor. Primal experiences that are relived during birth can be frightening to the mother as well as to those attendants who have little insight into or experience with this kind of psychodrama.

Many of the symptoms ascribed to the end of the dilation phase of labor ("transition") are no different from the signs of severe anxiety: sweating, trembling, nausea, shivering, and irritability. The involuntary shaking and trembling result from tension release in areas through which energy flow had been blocked. Self-regulated breathing alters with increased metabolic demands, stress, and effort. Thus, changes in a mother's breathing reflect the work being done by her body, as she breathes in energy and breathes out pain. The onslaught of the final dilating contractions is often perceived as relentless: The physical reality of fatigue leads to a lower pain threshold. It is easiest for the mother if she can tune in and surrender to each contraction. By allowing her breath to respond freely, noisy or otherwise, her labor can unfold without resistance. The natural amnesia of labor diminishes her sense of time and awareness of her surroundings.

Often the body's messages are extremely powerful and may demand an active response from the mother, such as strong rocking movements, heavy sighing, or loud groans. As her breath is linked to her emotions, it is essential that the mother not be discouraged from vocalization. Opening the mouth helps the uterus and vagina to open as well, deep sounds involve the diaphragm and relax the throat. All this may signal to attendants that the mother is "losing control," but she must ignore attendants' reactions and, like a swimmer, go with the waves, expressing herself however she wants.

Letting go in labor depends on a couple's level of self-control, a supportive birth environment (both emotionally and physically), and, most of all, respecting the natural rhythms of birth.

Some mothers experience a lull between the final wringing-out contractions that dilate the cervix and the onset of the urge to push with the expulsive force of the uterus. This pause, a time of peace and rest, is rarely observed or tolerated in hospitals. Pacing a birth according to hospital standards, rather than events of the birth itself, causes discomfort and disorients the mother from her body. Pushing that is forced by the staff and is too soon is a

No force of mind or body can drive a woman in labor, by patience only can the smooth force of Nature be followed.
GRANTLY DICK-READ

common occurrence, characteristic of institutional haste and active management of labor.

The Urge to Push

Women who have given birth before may experience the urge to bear down with the final dilating contractions, if the baby's head is low enough. A first-time mother may experience pressure of her baby's head against her rectum. If the head is still high in her pelvis, she may confuse this pressure with the expulsive urge.

Expectant parents usually do not understand the physiology of expulsion, and it is rarely explained to them. The expulsive urge is a natural reflex with which the uterus can engage the mother's assistance to help birth the baby. When the fetal head descends and stretches the pelvic floor, special nerve endings called proprioceptors are stimulated. These nerves carry the message to the pituitary gland in the brain, causing oxytocin to be released. (Another example of this neurohormonal reflex is nursing the baby to help expel the placenta. Breastfeeding also assists the uterus in shrinking back to its normal size through the release of oxytocin.)

Dr. Alois Vasicka of the North Central Bronx Hospital in New York found that natural oxytocin levels increase with the progress of second-stage labor, peaking when the baby's head crowns. Dr. Caldeyro-Barcia showed in his research how the "impulse" — the internal pressure of the uterine and abdominal muscles from contraction multiplied by the time interval during which the mother pushed — increased threefold by the end of the birth. Why are so many mothers made to push early on, when they have just completed cervical dilation, or criticized for not pushing effectively at this early time? Why the big hurry?

Occasionally, a mother may feel like pushing before her cervix is dilated, which as we have seen, relates to the descent (or "station") of her baby's head. If the urge is irresistible, the mother *cannot* hold back. Attendants who

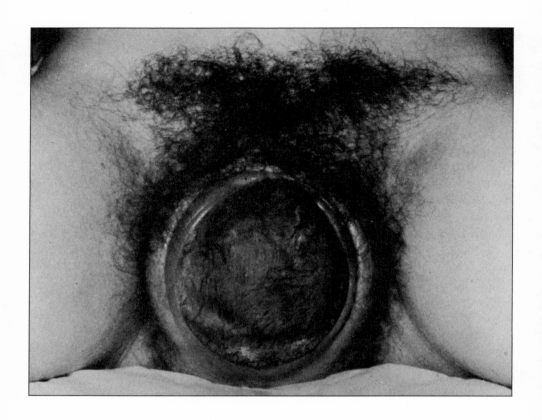

encourage her to continue with breathing patterns do so to no avail. A better guideline for attendants is that if it hurts a mother to push, she won't continue pushing voluntarily. If it feels right and good for her to push, then the mother will let her contraction sweep her along.

Because labor has been divided into artificial stages with fixed time limits, a small percentage of women are classified as having no urge to push. How much time was given for the mother's urge to become established? Where is the fetal head in relation to the pelvic floor? Helping the mother to assume an upright birth position such as squatting, stimulating her nipples, or stretching her vagina can be tried by attendants to bring on the expulsive urge (by increasing oxytocin output) if they are concerned with the delay. Sitting the mother on the toilet may help, as this (not the bed) is the place where she is accustomed to opening her pelvic muscles. Often contractions without an accompanying desire to bear down continue for over an hour. Then, just a couple of pushes may be needed once the baby's head reaches the perineum. Other mothers relax and let go so well that they give birth effortlessly; the uterus alone eases the baby out.

Any anesthesia, whether it is paracervical, pudendal, spinal, or epidural, abolishes this pushing reflex. Because sensory input from the muscles is removed by the anesthetic, falling oxytocin levels lead to weaker contractions. This is particularly so in the case of epidurals, as they are usually administered in the first stage of labor. Promoted to consumers as the "Cadillac of anesthesia," epidurals abolish sensation but not muscle power. However, the loss of sensation diminishes the oxytocin output so that forceps are frequently required. To avoid the need for instruments, some physicians do not replenish the anesthesia in second stage, so that it is allowed to wear off and contractions can pick up strength by the time of delivery.

Most women are not fully prepared for the increasing intensity of labor in second stage or for the climax of birth. Instead, they learn in prenatal class that after making it to the transition stage — the top of the mountain — all they will have to do then is follow the instructions of the staff. The doctor will tell the mother when to stop pushing and when to pant in order to restrain her urge to bear down. This allows the obstetrician to perform the delivery, rather than to let the mother give birth by herself.

Nursing students frequently ask me how to "develop techniques for spontaneous pushing." This is a contradiction in terms. Pushing is spontaneous. By definition, it is not done according to techniques! Women do not need to be taught how to push during birth any more than they need to be taught how to have an orgasm. Mothers learn, in labor, that pushing happens when the body is ready and the mind lets go. Breathing takes care of itself. The mother pushes out the baby with her exhaled breath, typically a grunt or a groan; partial closure of her glottis brakes her breath. Her abdominal muscles shorten most effectively on outward breath, and draw in, pressing on the uterus in the way that toothpaste is squeezed from a

Groaning is a way to release the diaphragm slowly and thus avoid extremes of tension. This is seen in the paraplegic, so it is not related to pain.
GRANTLY DICK-READ

tube. If a mother labors with insight, then her body can work effectively without undue exertion. Instead of using forceful techniques that consume energy, the mother can relax and wait for her baby to lead the way.

The spontaneous movements that occur during birth, like the sounds, are similar to those of female orgasm. Wilhelm Reich observed decades ago that any letting go of the breath and the body entailed a posture of surrender. The head glides back and the shoulders move forward and up. As the middle of the abdomen is drawn in, the pubic area moves upward and the legs spread apart. This natural opening up is most obvious in a reclining position. In contrast, the typical "managed" birth shows the posture of sexual armoring (tense shoulders and neck, rigid chest, breath held) that Reich observed and helped to release.

Unlike the Valsalva breathing maneuver, spontaneous pushing does not disturb physiology. Transient dips are observed in the fetal heart rate (see Appendix 4, page 124), but these are benign and associated with normal head compression during expulsive contractions. Dr. Caldeyro-Barcia found that the average number of pushes per contraction was four, and the average length of each push was four to five seconds. In contrast, couples have been taught in childbirth classes that the mother must hold her breath for three intervals of twenty seconds, as contractions last about a minute. Usually only a snatch breath is permitted. This contributes to the mother's hypoventilation. The natural intervals between spontaneous pushes prevent the fluctuations seen in the mother's blood pressure and the fetal heart rate when pushing is forced and prolonged.

Length of Second Stage of Labor

The duration of the expulsive phase of labor is of ongoing concern to physicians. As we have seen, the typical breath-holding and pushing results in slowing of the fetal heart rate and build-up of waste products in the fetal circulation. Doctors are anxious to deliver babies as quickly as possible, particularly if there is any fetal distress. However, often fetal distress is a result of the forced and prolonged pushing that the mother is obliged to do.

Instead of counting minutes or hours in second stage, we need to ask what the mother is doing. In homebirths, women often have second-stage labors that last for several hours but rarely does a mother physically push for all that time. We have seen that an interval usually passes between full dilation and the descent of the baby's head to the pelvic floor. If second stage were considered to begin at this point, then birth would be handled very differently by obstetricians.

Many skilled midwives count the onset of second stage when they can see the presenting part.
CHLOE FISHER

Another key factor in the length of second stage is the position of the occiput, which is the back of the baby's head leading the way out. Like the hands of a clock, the head may be lying in any position relative to the mother's pelvis. It is asymmetrical — facing either right or left — until just before the birth, then the head rotates to a front position. The usual and easier way of birth occurs when the occiput is anterior, or facing frontward toward the mother's pubic bones. However, in about a quarter of labors, the occiput is in the exact opposite or posterior position. Pressing against the mother's backbone, this bony prominence can cause constant "back labor" — backache that does not pass with the contraction. Because the head has to rotate so much farther around to bring the occiput under the pubic bones, such labors tend to be longer and more painful. Moving around a lot and assuming active, upright positions is often essential for the mother if such a labor is to progress without the need for instruments to rotate the head and deliver the baby. (See Appendix 5, page 125.)

Second stage, thus, can vary from a couple of pushes to *several* hours of hard work and pain. The shape of a mother's pelvis is another consideration, as the baby's head turns sideways to fit through the shape of her inlet and then straightens vertically to pass through the outlet. The relationship between the size of the baby's head and the space within the mother's pelvis is rarely the cause of a caesarean. The baby's skull bones are not fixed; they over-lap so the head can be molded to fit. Women who have had caesareans for so-called disproportion with their first baby often go on to deliver larger babies vaginally.

Haptonomic birth preparation, developed in France and the Netherlands, emphasizes contact between the parents and the child throughout labor. Frans Veldman feels that the purpose of contractions is to bring the baby's head symmetrically into the mother's pelvis so that the baby can then accomplish his or her birth. The father supports the mother from behind as she sits or squats. Placing his hands around her lower abdomen, he helps the mother keep her lower spine rounded and her pelvis tilted back. The outlet then faces forward and the baby is supported in a vertical position. The mother assists the baby's descent with gentle pressure on the baby's buttocks. In this way, both parents remain in physical and emotional contact with their child right through to the birth.

In his study on the physiological and psychological bases for the modern and humanized management of normal labor, Dr. Caldeyro-Barcia concluded that if the vital signs are normal, second stage does not have to be hurried. In his research, the outcome for the infants was excellent whether the expulsive phase of labor was brief or lasted over two hours. The blood gas results on the infants showed improved values over those currently recognized as normal, because there was no interference in any way with the natural process of labor. The unforced pushing efforts of short duration, avoiding the Valsalva maneuver and allowing ventilation of the lungs between pushes preserved normal physiology. The sitting position increased the mothers' comfort and enhanced the natural progress of labor. The women in his study had no sedatives, narcotics, anesthesia, or pitocin. The membranes were not artificially ruptured, which meant less pressure and molding of the baby's head. Finally, in the 1980s, it was proved that normal birth with no intervention is best for mother and baby!

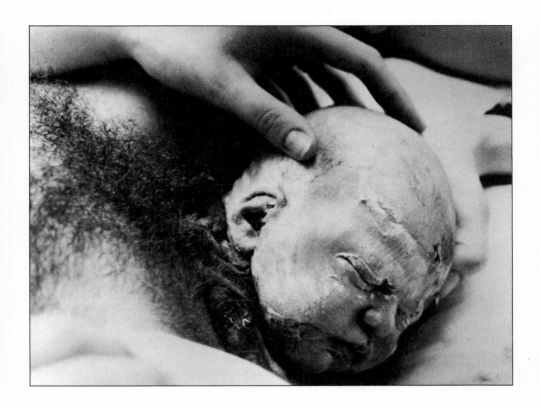

Birthing the Baby's Head

The resistance of the mother's pelvic tissues affects the progress of birth. If her muscles are tense or unsupple, they will not stretch easily. If her pelvic floor is anesthetized, then all tone is lost in the muscular "trough" that helps rotate the baby's head. When there is very little resistance to be overcome in her pelvic tissues, then the urge to push may not be strong at all, yet her baby may be born very quickly. Generally, the more times a woman gives birth, the less the resistance in her pelvic floor. By the same token, some doctors are worried that women can "overstrengthen" their pelvic floor muscles through ballet, horseback riding, or other exercise. Dr. Arnold Kegel has demonstrated in his film on the pelvic floor that it is the strong healthy muscle that stretches without injury. A weak, fibrous muscle is dragged down with the fetal head making tearing likely.

Oils, hot compresses, and manual support for the perineum are popular in alternative birth settings. While many attendants believe that these techniques help the perineum to remain intact, to be consistent with my concern about birth interference, I question whether this is natural or necessary if the mother is in an upright position and easing out the head with her own timing. Some perineums tear despite these protective measures. In many countries, midwives refrain from touching the perineum at all, with good results. Touch is a stimulus, and for some people a distraction that can create tension. Heavy pressure against the anus can actually cause the pelvic muscles to contract. Slipping a finger between the rim of the vagina and the baby's head to "iron out" the perineum takes up precious space. In the squatting position, it is difficult for the attendant to support (or cut!) the perineum. In the Curitiba, Brazil, clinic of Drs. Moyses and Claudio Paciornik, all births are done in the squatting position with no guarding of the perineum. Dr. Michel Odent also does not touch the perineum. Women who have experienced Haptonomic preparation can release both voluntary and involuntary tension in the perineum and thus offer no resistance to the baby.

A personal decision, then, has to be made by the attendant and the mother. Some attendants feel adamant that the perineum needs support; some mothers find the compresses very comforting and helpful in guiding the way they push. It certainly is a simple task to have a Crockpot of hot water handy. Expectant mothers need to be prepared for the sensations of vaginal stretching — stinging, burning, and finally numbness.

Psychological aspects are significant during crowning, especially the willingness with which a woman wants to receive her newborn. Some women want to be pregnant and love their fecundity, but they have not figured on the reality of birth and for some reason are afraid to see the child they have carried. Others suffer pregnancy just to be able to have the child they desire.

As the baby's head emerges from her body, the mother may reach down and feel it with her hands, lifting the

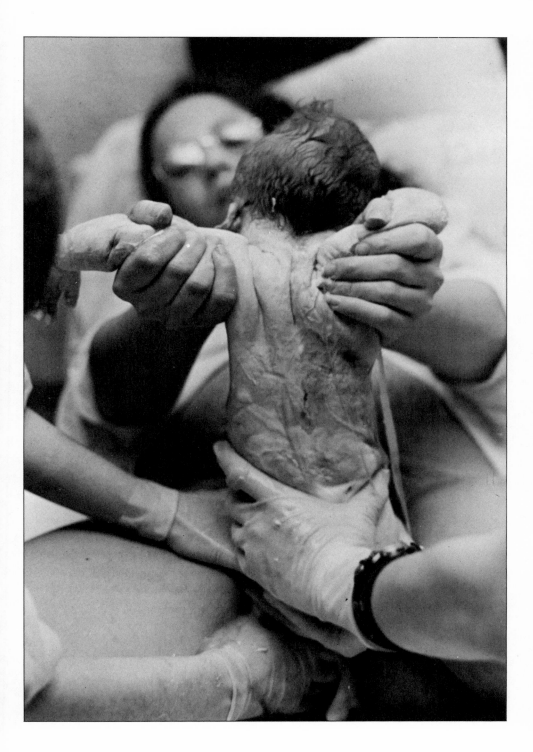

baby onto her body. If she is squatting or kneeling, she may just watch her baby for a couple of minutes before touching the baby. The mother's body heat keeps the baby warm, especially skin contact, when both are naked. Sometimes a baby, when placed on the mother's naked belly, will make crawling movements toward the nipple. Most will nurse at the breast right away. Breastfeeding facilitates expulsion of the placenta and membranes, which usually follow shortly after birth.

In ideal circumstances, the transition from the uterine existence to the parents' welcoming arms has gone smoothly for the baby. The powerful experience of birth stimulates the baby in preparation for the outside world, and newborns have striking, wide, alert eyes, which intensify the bonding process at this time. Fatigue from the physical work of labor seems to drop away, as the mother ecstatically greets the child she has grown to know and love in the preceding nine months. Together, the new family joyfully share in the miracle of life.

Resources

Books and Articles

HOSPITAL INTERVENTIONS

Annas, George J. *The Rights of Hospital Patients.* New York: Avon, 1975. An American Civil Liberties Union handbook covering informed consent, refusing treatment, organization of the hospital, medical records, confidentiality, and legal action. Written in an easy question-and-answer format.

Elkins, Valmai Howe. *The Rights of the Pregnant Parent.* Revised ed. New York: Two Continents, 1980. Tips for dealing with doctors and hospitals. (Skip the "Yankee Doodle" and controlled breathing.)

Haire, Doris. "How the FDA Determines the 'Safety' of Drugs — Just How Safe Is 'Safe'?" Available for $1 (includes postage) from the American Foundation for Maternal and Child Health, 30 Beekman Pl., New York, NY 10022. An exposé of the inadequacy of drug testing and evaluation.

DEVELOPMENT OF THE BABY

Flanagan, Geraldine. *The First Nine Months of Life.* Philadelphia: International Ideas, 1975. Black and white photographs of a baby's growth in the uterus. Good accompanying text.

Nilsson, Lennart. *A Child Is Born.* Revised Edition. New York: Delacorte, 1977. Classic color photographs showing how a baby develops in the uterus.

THE EXPERIENCE OF PREGNANCY AND BIRTH

Bittman, Sam, and Sue Rosenberg Zalk, Ph.D. *Expectant Fathers.* New York: Dutton, 1978. Explores a broad range of questions through pregnancy, birth, and early fatherhood. Emphasis on feelings and communication.

Brewer, Gail Sforza, ed. *The Pregnancy After 30 Workbook.* Emmaus, Penn.: Rodale Press, 1978. Recommended for women of any age. Excellent on nutrition and labor alternatives.

Colman, Arthur, and Libby Colman. *Pregnancy, The Psychological Experience.* New York: Bantam, 1975. Based on studies with pregnant women; describes characteristic emotions of expectant mothers and fathers during each trimester.

Hazell, Lester. *Commonsense Childbirth.* New York: Tower, 1975. Excellent general guide with sections on homebirth, breastfeeding, and unexpected outcome.

Kitzinger, Sheila. *The Experience of Childbirth.* 4th edition. New York: Penguin, 1978. The first and best book by this famous British childbirth educator. Emphasizes harmony of the body with feelings and emotions. (Ignore the controlled breathing.)

———. *Giving Birth: The Parents' Emotions in Childbirth.* New York: Schocken, 1977. Personal accounts expressing the individuality and range of birth experiences.

Lang, Raven. *Birth Book.* Palo Alto, CA: Genesis Press, 1972. Personal descriptions of homebirths, good instructions, and wonderful photographs.

Marzollo, Jean, ed. *9 Months, 1 Day, 1 Year: A Guide to Pregnancy, Birth and Baby Care, Written by Parents.* New York: Harper Colophon, 1976. A chronology of many expectant parents' views and feelings.

Meltzer, David. *Birth.* New York: Ballantine, 1981. A collection of myths, legends, poems, and essays.

Milinaire, Caterine. *Birth: Facts and Legends*. New York: Crown, 1974. Assorted accounts of different births and lifestyles. Information presented in a readable, personal style.

Wachstein, Alison E. *Pregnant Moments*. Dobbs Ferry, N.Y.: Morgan, 1979. Beautiful photos with good text.

Films

Five Women, Five Births. Suzanne Arms Productions, 151 Lytton Ave., Palo Alto, CA 94301. A film, in black and white stills, about women making choices. Home, hospital, and breech births.

The Squatting Position Delivery (8 mm and 16 mm). Polymorph Films, 118 South St., Boston, MA 02111. A brief, remarkable Brazilian film showing spontaneous unassisted births.

Kegel, Arnold, M.D. "The Pathological Physiology of the Pubo-Coccygeus Muscle in Women." Hollywood, Calif.: Morgan Camera Shop, 1953. Historic exploration of pelvic floor development, function, dysfunction, and rehabilitation through exercise. Very technical; recommended for medical audiences. Available for rental from Maternal and Child Health Center, 2464 Massachusetts Ave., Cambridge, MA 02140.

Slides

Dania's Birth (color). Suzanne Arms Productions, 151 Lytton Ave., Palo Alto, CA 94301. Moving story of a homebirth showing wonderful support from family members and midwives.

Welcome Emily! (black and white). Diane Gent, 3310 Green Rd., Beachwood, OH 44122. Family-centered birth in a homelike birth center. Difficult, noisy, realistic labor.

CHAPTER 5

Preparation for a Journey into the Unknown

BEFORE SETTING out on a journey into the unknown, any explorer takes care of practical considerations that may be reasonably anticipated. Likewise, expectant parents need to carefully shop around for birth attendants, gather supplies for a homebirth, or inspect maternity centers and hospitals to find an institutional birth environment that suits their needs and expectations.

Exploring Expectations of Birth

Expectant couples need to explore their hopes and fears as much as possible to avoid letdowns. Individual expectations are closely allied to personal goals. Goals lie in the future yet they often obscure the present. Students work years for degrees in fields where jobs no longer exist. Hardworking men and women often do not know how to spend their leisure time once they retire. The best laid plans continuously need to be reviewed and reshaped. What we expect is often not fully acknowledged until plans fail to materialize and we feel disappointment. Either pessimists or optimists, we rarely recognize both good and bad in our plans when we set goals.

Hope for the best, but plan for the worst.
PROVERB

Group discussion in childbirth classes helps to raise questions and force prospective parents to confront difficult matters. Some instructors encourage this by handing out cards with open-ended phrases to be completed, such as "What I dread most about having a baby . . ." and "The baby's arrival will affect our life by . . ." Dr. Leni Schwartz suggests that expectant parents take turns with the Gestalt game "I resent" and "I appreciate" to enhance their communication.

Ongoing prenatal exercise classes also enable a great amount of information to be shared by women, and the group offers support over several months for dealing with change and growth. Expectant mothers often share feelings in a group of women that they may not so readily express in front of couples.

It is my hope that fathers' psychological participation during pregnancy and birth will come to be seen increasingly as a source of personal gratification for men, and will not be something that is done simply to please their partners.
LENI SCHWARTZ

Individual and couple counseling is also very valuable. Unfortunately, the medical approach to prenatal care overlooks the psychological dimensions of pregnancy. Many pregnant women could be helped to confront difficulties they may be experiencing in the relationship they have with their partner, their parents, or other children. Pregnant women often find that suppressed memories of their own births may start to surface in the form of dreams — perhaps with images of being trapped in a locked house or clothes dryer or with the sensation of squeezing or pressure.

Fathers-to-be report more dreams during their partners' pregnancies, and show an increase in physical ailments, such as nausea, headaches, weight gain or loss. A father may feel envy or distaste toward his partner's pregnant body, along with decreased sexual satisfaction and fears that the mother's attention will be totally absorbed by their baby. The impending crisis of birth also forces an expectant father to review his own experience of being fathered and to create a behavior model for himself. In recent years, the psychological needs of fathers through the childbearing year have received much attention in books, films, and research studies.

During pregnancy, it is important for couples to expose themselves to the enormous range of birth experiences through books, slide shows, films, and discussions with new parents. Contact with newborn babies helps to ce-

teeth brush soap
11 Paste make up
nightgown
robe
clogs

yellow pads

Anita = students -

Paula -
Angela -   Singer

Mike - Hunter
        Hunger

1) nightgown
2) robe
3) slippers
   all
   Lynn

Purl and

4th -

6.00
3.50/88

ment a couple's realization that they, too, will soon be spending up to twenty-four hours a day caring for a total dependent.

Nutrition

We are what we eat. Diet is a good place for a pregnant woman to begin with (moderate) changes to help her expand her awareness of how different foods affect her feelings and behavior. Typically, expectant mothers may lose all taste for alcohol, caffeine, and tobacco, all of which have an adverse effect on nutrients as well as on a growing baby. Learning to observe dietary needs — developing nutrition through intuition — is a slow but rewarding process. After all, eating and drinking is something we do several times a day and is of interest to all of us.

A seeker once asked a Zen master how he knew he had attained enlightenment. "I eat when I am hungry and I drink when I am thirsty" was the reply.
PAUL REPS

While nutrition is full of controversies, pregnancy offers the chance to study and experiment with a diet that suits individual needs and taste while ensuring a healthy, normal birth-weight baby and a well-nourished mother. Nutrition is the most important aspect of prenatal care and the couple must take responsibility for seeing that the mother-to-be has an adequate and balanced daily intake of good food. (Recommended guides are found on page 113.)

Movement and Stretching

Exercise, along with sound nutrition, rest, and relaxation, is necessary for a healthy life. In less sedentary times, our daily existence took care of these needs. Nowadays, we have to make the time for calisthenics, yoga, jazzercise, golf — whatever.

Although everyone could benefit from a thorough examination of their muscles and joints, it is safe to say that certain groups of muscles need strengthening and others need stretching. Generally, people are more tense and tight than they are weak. Women, in particular childbearing women, can benefit from improving the power of the abdominal and pelvic floor muscles as described in my book *Essential Exercises for the Childbearing Year*.

Stretching involves extension, opening up, relaxation. It should be an integral part of every sport, dance, or exercise program, as well as of daily life. Stretching, one of the most enjoyable physical experiences, is commonly overlooked in favor of goal-oriented movements. Sixty sit-ups only look more impressive than bending forward with the legs astride!

Bioenergetics positions* are helpful to ground the energy in people who live mostly "in their heads." "Grounding" means letting energy move through the body center and pelvis to the legs. Pregnant women with poor circulation and cold feet benefit from grounding exercises. When people feel support beneath their feet, they experience their legs as strong yet flexible. As a result, they feel the courage to stand and move alone, in touch with reality. Specific examples of how to ground the body and free the breathing can be found in the books of Alexander Lowen, M.D.

Polarity Therapy also helps with energy distribution by balancing the negative and positive charges throughout the body through touch that can be active or passive.

Prenatal exercise classes make a woman aware of her balance, posture, strengths, and weaknesses. Also, any body work exposes one's physical and mental resistance to change. In the best prenatal classes, women are individually evaluated and exercise slowly and mindfully under careful supervision.

A program of physical activity should be comprehensive. For example a combination of calisthenic exercises that strengthen; stretching or yoga to ease out tight muscles; aerobics to improve the performance of the heart and lungs; and relaxation. Aerobics in pregnancy is more comfortable in nonweight-dependent positions that avoid stress on the pelvic floor and feet, such as swimming, cycling, ball games while seated, or movements on large gymnastic balls. Such a program encourages optimal

* The "bow" or backward bend in standing is unphysiological and should be avoided in the childbearing year.

strength, flexibility, coordination, and poise. The earlier a pregnant woman begins exercising, the better her health and comfort through the childbearing year. Exercise relieves stress and tension, creating a happier frame of mind.

As well as increasing limberness, stretching offers an opportunity to prepare for birth by *confronting pain and resistance*. Placing the body in various unaccustomed postures leads to distinct feelings of resistance and discomfort. By stretching to her limits — where it starts to hurt — and staying there, a woman can confront pain and look inward to her response. An amazing discovery follows. She will find that much of the pain relates to her fear of it. If she can accept the pain and dare to explore it — where and how it hurts, what type of pain she feels, what color it is — then the pain does not get worse, it actually diminishes. The same holds true for any unpleasant stimulus or extreme sensation, such as burn, itch, or cold.

We have two essential strategies for coping: the way of avoidance and the way of attention . . . The pain is the aversion; the healing magic is the attention.
MARILYN FERGUSON

Wanting to get out the pain is the pain.
ALAN WATTS

Stretching should be done gradually, with the assistance of gravity, and sustained for at least several seconds (ideally several minutes) while you slowly breathe and ease into it. It is beneficial if an expectant mother can sustain the stretch for one to two minutes — the approximate length of a contraction — to prepare for labor. She can repeat the experience as often as she is motivated and in countless ways. The more a person stretches, the more her muscles loosen and lengthen, and relaxation is gained from letting go. It is important always to stretch to one's limits, otherwise no challenge awaits the mind and no physical improvement occurs. To keep searching for a new area of resistance, another edge of pain, stretch farther or progress to a more advanced position. In this way, an expectant mother can actually pursue pain, on a level comparable to that of a labor contraction, which greatly improves her self-confidence and reduces her fear of her body and the birth.

Bouncing must always be avoided in stretching as this stimulates receptors that cause muscles to shorten instead of lengthen. Do not force yourself through the pain. Force only shuts down our consciousness of the process and all the small steps we are taking. A vigorous approach can lead to tendon injuries, especially in the pubic area and shoulders. It is important always to stretch both sides of the body; one side is usually less flexible than the other and requires extra attention and motivation.

The key to letting go is the natural flow of the breath, in and out, in and out. Anxiety from any threatening sensation causes tightness in the throat, tension in the body, and irregular breathing. To surrender to the body, to relax into positions or movements, the breath must be free to bring in energy and nourish the body. Tension in the throat or voice during labor is a sure sign of anxiety and the need for help to free the breath.

Stretching and holding postures calms the mind. Total concentration is involved. Positions involving balance also demand that our attention not wander. Yoga is the most well known discipline for stretching the body and mind, but a whole range of stretches can be found in *Stretching* by Bob Anderson. This book provides many preliminary and modified positions, so that a person at any level can get started. The *Runners' World Yoga Book* by Jean Couch and Nell Weaver is also helpful; it illustrates intermediate postures and the use of furniture for support.

Labor partners, especially men, can benefit from doing simple stretches in childbirth classes (such as back, hamstrings, shoulders). When they stretch to the point of pain, they can appreciate the sensations of labor (when first the cervix is stretched, and then the vagina) and understand the unity of mind and body. Generally, men are stronger but tighter physically. Individuals who are high achievers often cannot sit comfortably on the floor in a basic posture such as tailor-sitting. Flexibility is a condition of both body and mind and is affected by personality as much as by work habits or lifestyle.

Standing
loosen arms
neck
  breathflow
inbreathflow arms
  rising
softly to sides
as wings
opening
to fly.
PAUL REPS

Stillness of body creates quietness of breath; quietness of breath creates equanimity of mind, and equanimity of mind creates harmony of being.
JUDITH LASATER

Relaxation

As we saw in our discussion of the law of reversed effort (Chapter 3), immediate goals such as sleep, relaxation, or orgasm are just as elusive as long-term goals of destiny.

The more we try to attain, the more goals elude us. Some days we don't try as hard or don't expect to succeed, yet we are often pleasantly surprised that we fall asleep more easily or stretch farther than we anticipated.

Whenever we are self-conscious or afraid of failing, it seems almost inevitable that we make the very mistakes we want to avoid. Likewise, children who are told repeatedly not to drop something, invariably become clumsy. Intellectual programming for birth can fall flat because our expectations are set in the future and our feelings cannot be anticipated. *Preliminaries* is a term used by therapists to describe the beginning or intermediate levels of sensory or movement experience, while concern for a goal or instant result is set aside. The means — touching, looking, listening, feeling, holding a body position — rather than the ends (orgasm, talking, performing an exercise) are explored. Because fear of performance is removed, this approach has worked well in treating problems of stress in both men and women. The successful resolution of sexual difficulties through this approach has been described in *The Pleasure Bond* by William Masters and Virginia E. Johnson.

Relaxation is the key to awareness and energy. People who never relax only know tension, which feels unpleasant and interferes with many body functions. When the muscular system is unblocked and breathing flows freely, energy is liberated throughout the body. Letting go is blissful release when one has been tense. Women who have found ways to release tension in labor experience contractions as very different, almost pleasurable.

Scientists have documented beneficial changes that occur during a state of relaxation. Case histories bear witness to the tremendous healing powers we have within ourselves. Recent observations show that in a relaxed, dreamy state (the opposite of "control") there is an increase in endorphins, morphinelike substances secreted by the body that create euphoric feelings and raise the pain threshold. (We are usually more aware of the opposite phenomenon: how much worse pain feels when we are fatigued.) Reduction in muscle activity measured by bio-

We should not say "Relax!" but rather, "Why are you tense?"
EVA REICH

Contraction brings tension on the nerves; release brings freedom.
B. K. S. IYENGAR

feedback devices has shown changes in brain waves during relaxation or meditation. The presence of alpha wave patterns shows that relaxation is a different state of consciousness from sleep and full wakefulness.

Laura Mitchell, a British physical therapist, has written a useful guide aptly titled *Simple Relaxation.* Her approach offers an ideal replacement for "conscious release" exercises (see page 52). The basis of her instruction is a physiological law: the reciprocal relationship between opposite pairs of muscles. For example, when flexing your arm, the extensors must relax. Alternatively, when straightening your arm, the muscles that bend it must lengthen. Tension causes tightening and shortening of muscles. Characteristically, the flexor group predominates and tenses us for "fight or flight." Regardless of the source of the fear, anxiety, or stress, this pattern of muscular activity is always the same. The chest wall is rigid and breathing becomes impaired. Tense people typically sit with their legs and ankles crossed, arms folded, hands clenched, and shoulders hunched — a common sight!

We cannot will tight muscles to let go, because of the way that the nervous system works. Also the law of reversed effort requires our "passive volition." Mitchell, however, uses a fundamental principle in physical therapy: in order to coax a tight muscle to release, actively work its opponent. Relaxation is indirectly achieved through subtle movements of stretching, extending, opening. Actively *pulling* the shoulders *down* from the ears, for example, is different from raising or dropping them. The terminology in Mitchell's book is carefully chosen so that it is applicable in any position. Simple cues, such as "stretch the fingers long" or "drag down your jaw" are most useful during labor so a mother can quickly relieve tension where it concentrates.

Meditation means being in the present. Being in the present means letting go of what you think that present should be. This letting go is the process whereby one attains freedom.
JUDITH LASATER

Relaxation is a personal state and one that each of us has to explore for ourselves. To experience relaxation, couples need time, support, and freedom from judgment and competition. Instructors who move around in the room in prenatal classes, checking and comparing students' performances, often induce more stress than relaxation. There are many aids to help people relax, such as stretching, breath awareness, guided visualization, music, massage, hot baths or showers, and meditation.

Meditation encourages living in the here and now. Learning to keep thoughts in the present is the best way to let the future take care of itself, whether we are enjoying a stretch for the pleasure of stretching (and not just for the goal of achieving a certain flexibility), enjoying a pregnancy (without being preoccupied about what might happen in labor), or fully experiencing a contraction in labor (without worrying about the next one). Meditation practices include the use of breathing, mantras (meaningless sounds), chanting, and the use of candles and incense to expand the senses and limit thoughts. One of the more advanced skills in meditation involves the ability to "experience without naming," to have no separation between thinker and thought. Usually consciousness creates symbols that deflect our attention from the present moment with a series of judgments, depending on our attitudes.

Breath awareness is central to relaxation and meditation. In yogic lore a person's life span is predetermined by a certain number of breaths, therefore the slower and more efficiently one breathes, the longer one's life. Our breath links us with the universal energy and all living things. When we stop breathing, we die.

Because it is possible to become aware of one's breathing at any time, the nature of the breath is a handy gauge of tension levels in the body. Tense individuals have restricted breathing, leading to their lack of energy and vitality. Some people forcefully pull the abdominal wall in and out, as opposed to the natural rising and falling of the diaphragm. Others fix their diaphragms and raise their shoulders with each breath, causing neck tension and headaches. Becoming aware of one's breath helps one relax. The breathing becomes efficient and even, a balance of giving and receiving, expansion and contraction.

The breath can be used to quiet "mental chatter" and achieve a state of meditation. We can check which nostril is open, focus on how the chest and abdomen are moving, whether the breath is regular, or if there is a pause be-

Meditation is not a removal from relationship, but seeing oneself in relationship.
JOEL KRAMER

The meditator works much like the sculptor, removing the excess material so what lies hidden may be revealed.
SWAMI AJAYA

The easiest thing to do seems to us the hardest to let all self-imposed pressures of our nerve blood networks

To sit and look to sit and listen then to move interests us

Even more interesting may be to sit in one's given breathflow and let go with it friends of birds and clouds.
PAUL REPS

tween the exhaled breath and the subsequent inhalation. Deep relaxation occurs when you can let yourself be so passive that you feel as if you are being "breathed" by your body. As we become more sensitive to our breathing, we feel how it changes when certain thoughts enter our minds, or when we engage in certain activities. Even after a minute or so of controlled breathing, such as practicing a panting pattern for labor, it is surprising how long it takes for breathing to settle down to its own rhythm again. There is a world of difference between observing or attending to the breath and controlling it by altering the speed or depth.

The body is in the past, reflecting its tensions; the mind is in the future; and the breath is the only thing we have in the present. It is the basis of all meditation and conscious birthing.
JUDITH LASATER

Any control of the breath involves effort and causes tension. It is helpful to try various artificial breathing patterns that may be taught in childbirth classes and contrast these with letting the breath take care of itself. Also try breathing with the eyes open and then closed, and experiment with normal breathing and artificial patterns for labor while doing stretching exercises to the point of pain. As Doris Haire suggests to doubters, "Try controlling your breath from now until you go to bed tonight. You can breathe any way you like, but just make sure you control each breath." Most people are amazed to discover what an effort it is to control their breath, especially for long periods, and invariably prefer to let the breath go at its own pace. Allowing the breath to flow freely dissolves resistance in the body and enables a mother to yield to the contractions in labor. Of course, many changes will spontaneously occur in her breathing — reflecting her emotions, the intensity of her contractions, and the physical demands of her body at this active time.

Simply being seems boring because our awareness of our existence is so superficial, always looking forward to tomorrow.
ALAN WATTS

When experiencing breath awareness, let thoughts that arise just pass through your mind. Don't try to control them or block them out. Keep returning to the rhythm of your breathing. Allowing attention to flow with the breath quiets thinking, calms the emotions, and leads to physical release.

Vocalization. Breath awareness can be taken further into "sounding." Many women in labor are inhibited about noises they may make, although these usually occur spontaneously. Preparation for vocalization encourages women to make noise freely. This helps relieve tension during pregnancy as well as labor. Any blockage of feeling affects vocal expression and creates tension around the diaphragm, throat, and vocal apparatus. During the stress of labor, the breath is exhaled in a sigh, groan, grunt, or roar. If no sound is heard from a woman in labor, her breath may be blocked.

In Toning Therapy, exhale breathing is used to heal from the inside out. The voice releases the power in the body and helps shatter a negative condition. We all know that sound has external physical effects. A soprano voice may break a glass. Plant growth is affected by music and the flow of breast milk can be increased with soothing melodies. Babies do not like hard rock music. Neither do skunks, according to a farmer who successfully got rid of one with it. Our breathing and heart rate also respond to sound and vibration.

Pregnant women enjoy the in-class experience of sounding or toning as it echoes through a group. They notice how it relaxes their throats and gives them a renewed sense of vitality. Sounds with no associated verbal meaning (mantras), such as *ah* or *om*, may be used, or, for more vibration effect, words with several syllables. Chants or affirmations (positive statements about the mind, spirit, or body) are alternatives. While sounds are used to calm the mind, silence — the interval — is just as important for relaxation.

In Pithiviers, France, a form of singing known as *psychophonie* is used in childbirth preparation. Singing while working is common in many cultures. Singing helps to unite the energy of the group and keep everyone's breath flowing during exertion. Because it is an expansive activity, it promotes well-being and relaxation. In my prenatal classes, women share their favorite songs and lullabies — sometimes to begin the session, at other times as a prelude to relaxation. Unborn babies respond to music and their parents' voices. In *The Secret Life of the Unborn Child*, Dr. Thomas Verny notes that musicians have reported that they "knew" certain pieces of music sight unseen, and

For changing people's manners and altering their customs there is nothing better than music.
SHU CHING

later verified that their mothers had practiced those scores during pregnancy.

Massage is a valuable tool for helping people become aware of their bodies. People enjoy being touched — if they are touched in the right way. Very light touch is especially relaxing for mothers and babies. Not only can couples learn a lot about each other from exchanging massages, but pregnant women love to touch and compare each other's bodies in all-women exercise classes. In sharing massage, we learn to give as well as to receive.

Massage of the feet and hands as in Reflexology or Zone Therapy can benefit organs and systems within the body. Polarity Therapy uses touch to balance the body's energy field. The therapist acts as a conductor at certain points of the woman's body, progressing in an orderly sequence. This passive approach, being firmly in touch but demanding nothing, often brings immediate results; images, memories, feelings surface as the energy flow is liberated. Polarity Therapy can help right-brained expectant mothers shift their energy to the other side — their female and intuitive side — which is a highly beneficial preparation for birth. (Postpartum, Polarity treatment is very effective if the mother has had a caesarean or an episiotomy. Such surgical trauma may result in dissociation from pelvic awareness, especially sexual feelings, and energy disturbances such as weakness in the knees. A couple of Polarity sessions can resolve these problems.)

Revitalizing the Dead Zones

All human experience takes place in the body, especially emotions such as fear. A person expresses him- or herself in every action or movement. But certain areas of our bodies become cut off from consciousness as we react to the customs and pressures of our environments. For example, most of us feel very awkward squatting. Shortening of muscles and stiffening of joints will not permit most of us to assume the squat position easily and correctly. However, as children we squatted naturally.

The first response to touch is always a response in breathing, through which one's vulnerability is disclosed.
FRANS VELDMAN

Childhood development springs from moving and feeling. Touch is the foundation for all the other senses and is at the seat of human feelings, emotions, and awareness. Most people have lost touch with sensations from joints and muscles. Because vision is such a conscious and dominant activity, few people can do movements well with their eyes closed, especially in a standing position.

Every disturbance of the ability to fully experience one's own body damages self-confidence as well as the unity of body feeling.
WILHELM REICH

While each person has to find her or his body's own dead zones, certain areas are typically neglected.* The trunk, especially the abdomen and pelvis, are usually zones of lower awareness than the arms or legs. Neurologically, there is a difference that relates to sensitivity and not size, in representation of body areas in the brain. Thus the feet, hands, and lips have a much richer network of nerves than, say, the small of the back. Sex organs are another very sensitive area, but they are isolated by the surrounding dead (in most people) pelvis, which causes sexuality to be experienced in a limited genital form, a release of tension rather than an experience of pleasure.

Wilhelm Reich observed that when his patients were able to let go within the pelvis, it had a liberating effect on their personalities as well. Holding back in the pelvis can result in chronic constipation, which leads to undesirable straining. Lack of pelvic awareness corresponds with diminished pelvic mobility. Some women may accept such inflexibility because pelvic movements are sexual and this makes them feel uncomfortable. The "pelvic clock" exercise described by Moshe Feldenkrais in *Awareness Through Movement* is a good place to begin. Belly-dancing is another way to focus on the pelvis. A great number of women cannot identify their pelvic floor muscles, or else these internal muscles are so weak that they barely contract.

The feet and lower legs are common dead zones. Grounding exercises elicit a sense of being connected throughout the whole body and help the feet to ade-

---

* The Haptonomic principles of touch develop from the sacral area of the pelvis. A person's awareness of his or her "base" is the key to emotional and physical security. Frans Veldman feels that a baby, from the moment of birth, should be picked up and carried from the base and that the head should never be touched. If the baby is held correctly from below, the head does not need support.

quately support and share the body weight. The arches of the feet, both long and transverse, are often flattened in pregnancy and give rise to foot pain. It can take several weeks before awareness and control of the small muscles of the feet are developed to improve arch support.

The neck, like the pelvis, is a bridge linking the mind with the body. Stiffness of the neck can affect posture. Chronic tension of the neck muscles gives rise to headaches, which ironically may occur when the muscles start to relax and the circulation starts to flood the tissues. The muscles then tense up in opposition, which perpetuates the vicious circle. Likewise, in other areas of the body, tingling, trembling, shaking, and other involuntary and unpleasant sensations may occur with the release of long-bound tension.

Dead zones can be worked on through a whole variety of approaches: stretching, massage, Haptonomy, biofeedback, Bioenergetics, Polarity Therapy, yoga, Feldenkrais method, Alexander technique, Trager system, EST, Rolfing, and visualization.

Visualization, in contrast to physical approaches to personal awareness, is a way to use the mind to visit the body. It is always useful to create hypothetical situations to help learn how to deal with fear. When pregnant, women enjoy a more fluid, suggestible state of mind than at other times in their lives. They can create rich images of the unborn baby, their inner organs, and the energy and opening up involved in birth. Visualization during actual contractions can be very helpful, too.

Gayle Peterson, a psychotherapist in Berkeley, California, specializes in visualization training for pregnant women, guiding them toward a positive birth experience utilizing hypnotic suggestion. Her approach has been successful in enhancing the normal process of labor, and has helped to resolve problems such as breech position of the baby. Skilled counseling can help pregnant women express their deepest feelings, even if this requires a regression back to their own infancies and births. Unfortunately, few childbirth educators are aware of the significance of these past experiences or of the therapeutic effect that reliving them brings about. Even fewer people teaching prepared childbirth have a background or interest in psychology, Haptonomic touch, Psychosynthesis, Gestalt, Bioenergetics, Primal Therapy, Rebirthing, or other ways to bring people to confront these experiences deep within themselves.

Although some emotional layers can be peeled off in group encounters, it takes time and one-to-one counseling to release buried feelings and primal pain. While practical considerations limit widespread application of this kind of psychotherapy,* it nevertheless remains of significant value. Childbearing is a time of personal crisis, when defenses break down and unresolved feelings emerge. Women in the most favorable of settings, such as at home with midwives, still may develop complications in their labors. This only proves the many hidden and complex levels on which our minds and bodies interact. Each birth has its own psychodrama and is a microcosm of a woman's entire life, beginning with her own conception.

Clear the surface so that growth can occur from the depths.
ALAN WATTS

Self-Acceptance

Expectant parents and childbirth educators can draw on a number of approaches to integrate the psychological and physical selves. It is beyond the scope of this book to discuss all the possibilities. An excellent guide is *In Our Own Hands* by Sheila Ernst and Lucy Goodison, who were members of a women's self-help therapy group. The book describes all the well-known therapies and personal growth strategies, with enough exercises to last a lifetime.

Learning situations should be pleasurable and easy, so that the breathing stays normal and the body wants to repeat the experience. Self-exploration is a matter of doing less but experiencing more. As a person's sensitivity increases, less effort is required and energy can be con-

To the extent that ability increases, the need for conscious efforts of the will decreases.
MOSHE FELDENKRAIS

* The terms *psychotherapy* and *patient* have negative connotations for many people. Some therapies, such as Radix, prefer to use the terms *education in feeling and purpose* and *student*. *Psychotechnology*, another new term, refers to the various approaches of the human potential movement that are intended to bring about a definite change in consciousness.

Letting myself feel vulnerable was my personal task. It was the first time I could let myself do it. I prided myself on my great strength before out in the man's world. I feel that to be a key issue in the contemporary world — allowing the feelings of vulnerability to be there instead of being in control and invulnerable. Surrendering, that's what one learns in therapy or I did anyway . . . allowing oneself to be sad, to be in pain, to feel fear . . . it's all part of life. "Anne," in The World of the Unborn *by* LENI SCHWARTZ

served, leading to heightened awareness. As sense perception becomes more acute, mind and body together become more dynamic and flexible, improving one's self-image.

If an adult is to change and grow, he or she needs to allow self-acceptance, without reservation. In pregnancy, especially, there is commonly a desire to be independent and responsible, yet at the same time to be nurtured and taken care of. Such ambivalence is characteristic of any major life transition. Some expectant mothers see themselves as very strong and superior to other women. They are often compulsive about their bodies and dismiss the value of relaxation and awareness, wanting to "work out" as hard as possible. It is possible to spot the fear behind this facade. With the right approach, usually quiet touch, their defenses dissolve and these mothers open up to their true selves. During the crisis of birth, all women need understanding, love, and support. In *Breastfeeding: The Tender Gift* Dana Raphael notes that successful nursing depends on the mother being mothered. (In other countries, e.g., Guatemala, the person, usually female, who provides that support is known as the *doula*. In the United States, the doula is most often the husband.)

Making Contact with the Unborn Child

Birth is an end and a beginning. Preparation for the journey into parenthood begins, ideally, well before the birth itself. Otherwise it can take some time for a mother to feel that her child belongs to her, even with the most auspicious of births. Inner bonding with the baby can happen only if an expectant mother bonds with her own body. As her unborn child is part of her body, a pregnant woman understands her child as well as she understands herself. How well she senses the child's feelings depends on how well she senses her own feelings.

Americans are astounded when they observe women in other cultures who carry their infants on their backs, without diapers, and without accidents. These women find it equally astounding to be asked how they know when their babies are ready to pass body wastes. They may often retort, "How do *you* know when you have to go?"

While some pregnant women see only a bulging belly, others are intimately connected with their unborn babies. Such women don't just go swimming, for example, they "take the baby swimming." They choose movements and music that they know their babies enjoy, and often set aside certain periods during the day to interact with their babies. Meditations, singing, conversation, prayers, stroking the belly, and patting any moving limbs are all part of the prenatal bonding process. The father can share in this communication, and the newborn will recognize his voice after birth. Many expectant couples sleep skin to skin so that the father can feel the baby's movement. Other suggestions to help couples get in touch with the baby can be found in *The World of the Unborn* by Leni Schwartz, and her cassette tape, *The Child Within*.

The baby's sense of self is believed to develop by about the sixth month of pregnancy according to research cited by Dr. Thomas Verny, author of *The Secret Life of the Unborn Child*. By birth, an infant is a very complex being. The unborn child senses a mother's continuing negative emotions, anxiety, or lack of love. Depression can originate in the uterus and newborns have died from peptic ulcers. Dr. Verny quotes one case of a baby who would breastfeed from other women but not from his own mother. All of a baby's experiences in the uterus are filtered through the mother. Clearly, her diet, peace of mind, and happy union with the unborn child are crucial.

Dreams, images, and intuitions help to provide a mother with insights into the personality of her unborn child. Some parental premonitions can be very accurate about the timing of birth, or detail about the labor or baby. *Born to Live* by Gladys McGarey, M.D., contains many unusual anecdotes of transpersonal prenatal experiences, strange coincidences, and miraculous healings, stressing the spiritual aspects of childbearing.

Simplifying Childbirth Preparation

In carrying on my own humble creative effort, I depend greatly on that which I do not know and upon that which I have not yet done.
MAX WEBER

The way to do is to be.
LAO TZU

Both childbirth educators and expectant couples can be relieved of a lot of pressure if prenatal classes are simple and flexible, emphasizing intuitive learning rather than role-learning. Attempts to use the mind to block messages from the body are philosophically, physically, and psychologically misconceived. As Alan Watts noted, this is like using the mind to get beyond the mind, using a mirror to reflect its own image, or using the eyes to see themselves. People need to integrate their minds and bodies, not to increase whatever division may exist between them.

Preparing for childbirth with insight means an expectant couple need no longer worry about staying "on top" of contractions or about controlling the uncontrollable events of birth. Instead, they can tune into each other and into the labor as it unfolds. Accepting intermittent pain, the mother will offer little resistance to it but flow with her breath and energy. Her partner, instead of consulting a stopwatch and printed outline of labor stages, carefully observes the mother's needs and provides her with comfort and reassurance. Helping her body to do its work as efficiently as possible, the partner assists the mother into various positions and movements of her choice. During the intensely powerful contractions, rather than concerning himself with how she is behaving or controlling herself, he offers his support to sustain her courage. Acknowledging her emotions, pain, and effort, he encourages her to stay in present time and to avoid judging her performance of the progress of the labor. As the baby's head and body emerge, both parents are joyfully united in the miracle of birth. They respond spontaneously to the events in ways that suit them as individuals and as a couple.

The role of the childbirth educator is to provide expectant couples with information for their minds and experiences for their bodies. A short course on obstetrics is necessary, as well as one on hospital labor procedures and alternatives. Facts about complications during labor and delivery may be more reassuring than threatening, although too much detail may actually increase complications by giving power to thoughts about them. Often couples learn that the incidence of problems is less than they had been led to believe by the medical profession and media. The need for informed consent during pregnancy or labor needs to be explained along with understanding the Pregnant Patient's Bill of Rights and Responsibilities. (See Appendix 6, page 126.) Skills for dealing with the hospital staff, such as decision-making and assertiveness training, should be developed in prenatal classes. A couple must make their needs known so that doctors and hospitals can be supportive — at least to some of those needs. (See the sample Birth Plan, Appendix 7, page 132.)

Preparation for childbirth ideally strengthens couples' self-reliance so they won't fall victim to the props of labor, be these drugs, fetal monitors, or temporary rescue measures such as distraction techniques and breathing patterns that promise control over the uncontrollable. The importance of group discussion and sharing to develop emotional security in facing uncertainty cannot be stressed too heavily. Couples themselves bring many resources to birth and may find ways of coping with pain, fear, and the unknown that instructors never considered.

The sexual, instinctual, and inevitable character of human birth must be conveyed to expectant couples. Listening to tape-recorded sounds of labor in the dark is a very powerful and moving experience. The spontaneous breath changes, cries, groans, grunts, and drawn-out pushes of different labors all help to show the power of contractions and the active surrender of the mother. Films or slides of naked birthing women depict birth as the sensual experience it is — the raw and naked force of nature. Although nakedness and noise are not encouraged in a hospital, such sights and sounds of labor help to sanction a woman's letting her body go where the contraction takes her, with no concern for outsiders' "standards of control."

The physical preparation through exercise and relaxation that an expectant mother experiences during pregnancy builds her self-confidence. If her labor is long and

Individual sexual instincts do not function independently of one another but form a unity as a liquid in connecting pipes. There can be only one uniform sexual energy which seeks gratification in various erogenous zones and psychic ideas.
WILHELM REICH

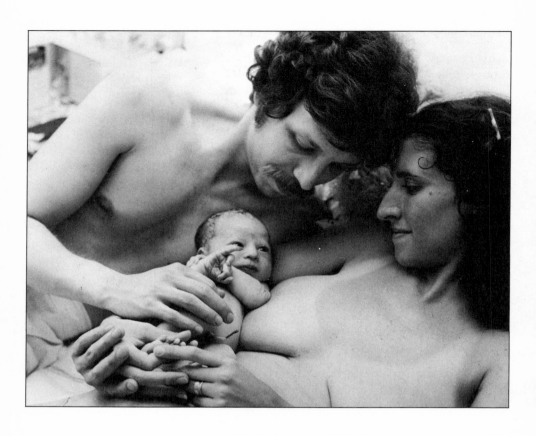

arduous, such preparation provides stamina and endurance. Physical self-discovery through stretching shows a woman where she is tight, and how she has to let go into the pain before she can open up. A birthing woman's role is to work with her body by relaxing deep inside herself and letting her labor happen. Frequently, the loss of energy is more of a problem in labor than the presence of pain. The more sensitive a woman is to her body's rhythms, the less energy she will expend during labor. Her active contribution will be guided by her contractions.

Expectant parents need to develop a sense of wonder as they embark on their birth journey into uncharted territory. With faith and courage, birth has the potential to be a peak experience, even if there are some difficulties and disappointments. The confidence that couples gain through a positive pregnancy and birth experience enables them to raise their child with self-assurance, depending

The mystery of life is not a problem to be solved but a reality to be experienced.
ALAN WATTS

less on professionals and outside experts. Confident parents trust their natural responses and exercise common sense. Parents today know that it is all right — even essential — to comfort a crying baby, and that all infants' stomachs are not designed for hospital feeding schedules. Mothers and fathers today are reclaiming their babies and carrying them on their bodies, feeding them at their breasts again, and sleeping with them in their beds. Women need to reclaim their birth experiences by trusting in the wisdom of nature and their bodies, and by laboring in their own individual ways. Birth, like love, is an energy and a process, happening within a relationship. Both unfold with their own timing, with a uniqueness that can never be anticipated, with a power that can never be controlled, but with an exquisite mystery to be appreciated.

Resources

Books

NUTRITION

Ballentine, Rudolph, M.D. *Diet and Nutrition.* Honesdale, Penn.: Himalayan International Institute, 1978. A fascinating overview of nutrition, covering both Eastern and Western views.

Brewer, Gail Sforza, with Tom Brewer, M.D., Consultant. *What Every Pregnant Woman Should Know: The Truth About Diet and Drugs in Pregnancy.* New York: Penguin, 1979. The importance of good nutrition in preventing toxemia in pregnancy; discussion of harmful dietary advice; includes recipes.

Williams, Phyllis. *Nourishing Your Unborn Child.* New York: Avon, 1975. Guide for pregnancy and postpartum, stressing natural foods; menus and recipes included.

Nutritive Value of Foods. Home and Garden Bulletin, #72. Available from: Science and Education Administration, U.S. Department of Agriculture, U.S. Government Printing Office, Washington, DC 20402. Analyzes common foods according to protein, fat, carbohydrate, vitamins, minerals and other nutrients. Resource for calculating dietary requirements.

STRETCHING

Anderson, Bob, with Jean Anderson. *Stretching*. Revised Edition. Bolinas, Calif.: Shelter Publications, 1980. An excellent and well-illustrated guide for men and women. Includes positions for all ranges of flexibility.

Couch, Jean, with Nell Weaver. *Runners' World Yoga Book*. Mountain View, Calif.: Anderson World, Inc., 1979. A clear guide to stretching and yoga, illustrating intermediate positions and helpful use of furniture.

RELAXATION

Keyes, Laurel Elizabeth. *Toning: The Creative Power of the Voice*. Marina Del Rey, Calif.: De Corss and Co., 1973. Making sounds for stress release, energy liberation, and healing. Cassette tapes are available from: Gentle Living Publications, 2168 S. Lafayette St., Denver, CO 80210.

Mitchell, Laura. *Simple Relaxation*. New York: Atheneum, 1979. Explains typical patterns of tension and simple stretches for release. Suggestions for pregnancy, birth, driving, and illness, etc.

White, John, and James Fadiman, eds. *Relax: How You Can Feel Better, Reduce Stress and Overcome Tension*. New York: Dell, 1976. Extensive overview of all relaxation methods with excerpts from different authors.

MASSAGE

Bergson, Anika, and Vladimir Tuchak. *Zone Therapy*. New York: Pinnacle, 1974. Detailed guide to foot and hand reflexology for diagnosing and treating other parts of the body.

Downing, George. *The Massage Book*. New York and Berkeley: Random House and the Bookworks, 1972. Basic guide to a wide range of massage techniques.

Gordon, Richard. *Your Healing Hands*. Santa Cruz, Calif.: Unity Press, 1978. A basic, illustrated introduction to Polarity Therapy.

SEXUALITY

Bing, Elisabeth, and Libby Colman. *Making Love During Pregnancy*. New York: Bantam, 1977. Sensitive and beautifully illustrated.

Masters, William H., and Virginia E. Johnson. *The Pleasure Bond: A New Look at Sexuality and Commitment*. New York: Bantam, 1976. Nonjudgmental examination of social and psychological aspects of sexual behavior.

MEDITATION AND VISUALIZATION

Swami Ajaya. *Yoga Psychology: A Practical Guide to Meditation*. Honesdale, Penn.: Himalayan International Institute, 1976. Describes the need for meditation, use in daily life, practical techniques.

Bry, Adelaide, with Marjorie Blair. *Visualization: Directing the Movies of Your Mind*. New York: Harper and Row, 1978. Many uses and practices of visualization for self-awareness and development.

Downing, George. *Massage and Meditation*. New York: Random House, 1974. Suggestions for breath exploration and visualizations for use with massage.

Gawain, Shakti. *Creative Visualization*. Mill Valley, Calif.: Whatever Press, 1978. Guide to growth of the imagination and spiritual development. Selected meditations, affirmations, goal-setting, and clearing exercises.

Peterson, Gayle H. *Birthing Normally: A Personal Growth Approach to Childbirth*. Berkeley, Calif.: Mindbody Press, 1981. Birth visualizations for childbirth educators to use with expectant parents. Very interesting case histories.

Samuels, Michael, and Nancy Samuels. *Seeing with the Mind's Eye*. New York and Berkeley: Random House and the Bookworks, 1975. Explains how visualization works; many techniques and exercises.

Schwartz, Leni. *The World of the Unborn*. New York: Richard Marek, 1980. Case histories of a pregnant couples' support group. Over forty ways to explore the emotions of pregnancy and communicating with the unborn.

AWARENESS AND GROWTH

Ernst, Sheila, and Lucy Goodison. *In Our Own Hands: A Woman's Self-Help Therapy*. Los Angeles: Tarcher, 1981. Very instructive and comprehensive book for self-exploration. Feminist stance. All kinds of individual and group exercises drawn from all major therapies.

Feldenkrais, Moshe. *Awareness Through Movement: Health Exercises for Personal Growth*. New York: Harper and Row, 1972. Clear explanation of human development with twelve practical lessons.

Lowen, Alexander, M.D. *Bioenergetics*. New York: Penguin, 1975. Describes how the body functions energetically and how to release muscular tensions.

Morningstar, Jim, Ph.D. *Spiritual Psychology*. Available from the author at 2728 N. Prospect Ave., Milwaukee, WI 53211. A holistic workbook dealing with mental and physical aspects of personal growth. Questionnaires, essay topics, and affirmations.

Stevens, John O. *Awareness: Exploring, Experimenting, Experiencing*. New York: Bantam, 1973. Over a hundred ways to expand personal and social awareness based on Gestalt therapy.

Williams, Strephon Kaplan. *Jungian-Senoi Dreamwork Manual*. Revised Edition. Berkeley, Calif.: Journey Press, 1980. A unique, detailed guide to exploring the unconscious through dreams.

GRIEVING

Borg, Susan O., and Judith Lasker. *When Pregnancy Fails: Families Coping with Miscarriage, Stillbirth, and Infant Death*. Boston: Beacon Press, 1981. A valuable guide to help family members of all ages work through grief and anger.

Klaus, Marshall H., and John H. Kennell. *Parent-Infant Bonding*, Revised Edition. St. Louis: Mosby, 1982. A revision and expansion of the original pioneering studies on human attachment to the newborn. Helpful chapters on coping with prematurity, malformation, and infant death.

BREASTFEEDING

Brewster, Dorothy Patricia. *You Can Breastfeed Your Baby . . . Even in Special Situations*. Emmaus, Penn.: Rodale Press, 1979. A thorough, well-illustrated reference for situations such as multiple births, prematurity, surgery.

Pryor, Karen. *Nursing Your Baby*. New York: Pocket, 1976. A practical guide for all aspects of breastfeeding.

Raphael, Dana. *Breastfeeding: The Tender Gift*. New York: Schocken, 1977. Describes the support and nurturing necessary for a mother to successfully breastfeed.

CARING FOR THE BABY AND BEING A PARENT

Brazelton, T. Berry. *On Becoming a Family: The Growth of Attachment.* New York: Delacorte, 1981. A supportive book to help parents stay in love with their babies. Excellent explanations of newborn behavior; many interesting family histories.

Brewer, Gail Sforza, and Janice Presser Greene. *Right from the Start: Meeting the Challenge of Mothering Your Unborn and Newborn Child.* Emmaus, Penn.: Rodale Press, 1981. Sound advice for the immediate postpartum, plus an excellent section on avoiding intervention during labor and birth.

Friedland, Ronnie, and Carol Kort, eds. *The Mothers' Book.* Boston: Houghton Mifflin, 1981. Candid personal accounts by mothers on the emotional aspects of parenthood. Wonderful, varied reading. Covers everything from pregnancy to triplets to single mothers to death.

Jones, Sandy. *To Love a Baby.* Boston: Houghton Mifflin, 1981. A poetic message, with beautiful photographs, exploring parental emotions and attachment to the unborn and newborn baby. Comprehensive annotated bibliography.

Montagu, Ashley. *Touching: The Human Significance of the Skin.* Revised Edition. New York: Perennial, 1978. An anthropological view of physical intimacy within families, child-raising practices. Discusses swaddling, rocking, breastfeeding.

Thevenin, Tine. *The Family Bed: An Age Old Concept in Childrearing.* Available from the author at P.O. Box 16004, Minneapolis, MN 55416. A convincing argument for families' sleeping together.

Wallerstein, Edward. *Circumcision: An American Health Fallacy.* New York: Springer, 1980. Thoroughly researched investigation into the medically unnecessary practice of circumcision.

Tape

Schwartz, Leni. *The Child Within.* Available from Leni Schwartz, 197 Oakdale, Mill Valley, CA 94941. A cassette of guided meditations and music for expectant couples.

Music

Lullabye from the Womb. Dr. Hajimi Murooka. Capitol Records ST 11421, 1974. Sounds of the mother's heartbeat and circulation, plus music to relax mother, unborn, or newborn.

Music for the New Age. Vital Body Marketing, P.O. Box 703, Fresh Meadows, NY 11365. Over two hundred records and tapes, Eastern and Western, for relaxation and meditation.

Narada Distributing, 1804 E. North Ave., Milwaukee, WI 53202. More than four hundred and fifty records and tapes of new-age music.

Organizations

La Leche League International, 9616 Minneapolis Avenue, Franklin Park, IL 60131. A volunteer organization of mothers with local chapters throughout the U.S. offering support and counseling for breastfeeding. Information pamphlets and nursing aids.

*Appendixes
Bibliography
Authorities Quoted*

Straining with the breath held for 20 seconds causes fluctuations
of the mother's blood pressure, excessive pressure in the uterus,
and slowing of the fetal heart rate.

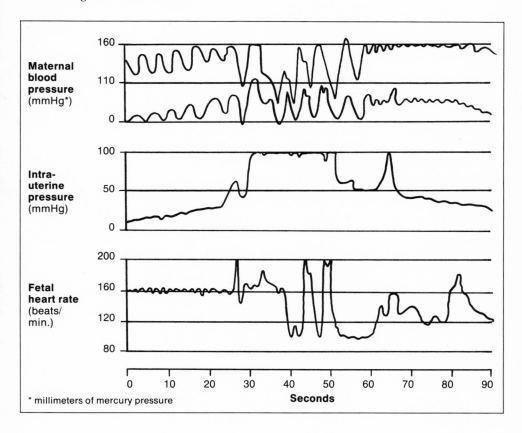

Contractions are more efficient and labor is shorter when the mother is propped in the upright position.

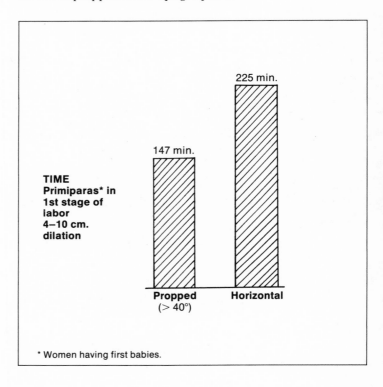

TIME
Primiparas* in
1st stage of
labor
4–10 cm.
dilation

147 min.

225 min.

Propped
(> 40°)

Horizontal

* Women having first babies.

An upright position of the mother widens the drive angle of the uterus and improves the progress of labor.

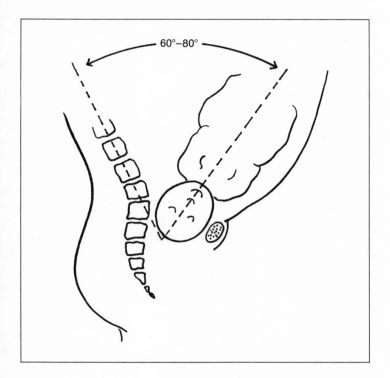

Spontaneous pushes occur several times in a contraction, last an average of only 4 to 5 seconds, and have a benign effect on the baby's heart rate.

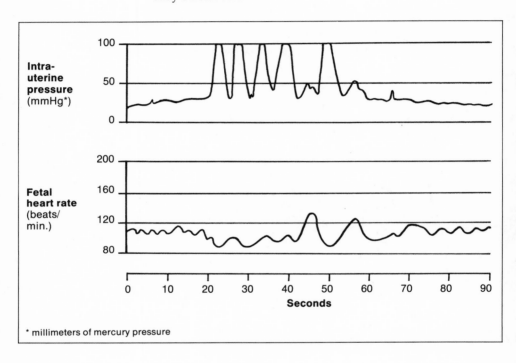

Intra-
uterine
pressure
(mmHg*)

Fetal
heart rate
(beats/
min.)

Seconds

* millimeters of mercury pressure

The fetal head rotates to fit through the contours of the pelvis. The inlet has its widest diameter horizontally and the presenting part of the head (occiput) is usually angled to the left or right side of the mother in a forward (anterior) direction or sometimes in a backward (posterior) direction. The occiput turns to an anterior position to pass through the pelvic outlet, which has its widest diameter vertically.

Pelvic Inlet: Baby's entrance

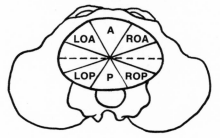

Pelvic Outlet: Baby's exit

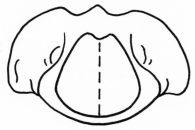

A = anterior (front)
P = posterior (back)
ROA = right occiput anterior (back of baby's head toward mother's right front)
LOA = left occiput anterior (back of baby's head toward mother's left front)
ROP = right occiput posterior (back of baby's head toward mother's right back)
LOP = left occiput posterior (back of baby's head toward mother's left back)

The Pregnant Patient's Bill of Rights

Prepared by Doris Haire, Chairperson of Committee on Health Law and Regulation, International Childbirth Education Association, Inc.

American parents are becoming increasingly aware that well-intentioned health professionals do not always have scientific data to support common American obstetrical practices and that many of these practices are carried out primarily because they are part of medical and hospital tradition. In the last forty years many artificial practices have been introduced which have changed childbirth from a physiological event to a very complicated medical procedure in which all kinds of drugs are used and procedures carried out, sometimes unnecessarily, and many of them potentially damaging for the baby and even for the mother. A growing body of research makes it alarmingly clear that every aspect of traditional American hospital care during labor and delivery must now be questioned as to its possible effect on the future well-being of both the obstetric patient and her unborn child.

One in every 35 children born in the United States today will eventually be diagnosed as retarded; in 75% of these cases there is no familial or genetic predisposing factor. One in every 10 to 17 children has been found to have some form of brain dysfunction or learning disability requiring special treatment. Such statistics are not confined to the lower socioeconomic group but cut across all segments of American society.

New concerns are being raised by childbearing women because no one knows what degree of oxygen depletion, head compression, or traction by forceps the unborn or newborn infant can tolerate before that child sustains permanent brain damage or dysfunction. The recent findings regarding the cancer-related drug diethylstilbestrol have alerted the public to the fact that neither the approval of a drug by the U.S. Food and Drug Administration nor the fact that a drug is prescribed by a physician serves as a guarantee that a drug or medication is safe for the mother or her unborn child. In fact, the American Academy of Pediatrics' Committee on Drugs has recently stated that there is no drug, whether prescription or over-the-counter remedy, which has been proven safe for the unborn child.

The Pregnant Patient has the right to participate in decisions involving her well-being and that of her unborn child, unless there is a clearcut medical emergency that prevents her participation. In addition to the rights set forth in the American Hospital Association's "Patient's Bill of Rights" (which has also been adopted by the New York City Department of Health), the Pregnant Patient, because she represents TWO patients rather than one, should be recognized as having the additional rights listed below.

1. *The Pregnant Patient has the right,* prior to the administration of any drug or procedure, to be informed by the health professional caring for her of any potential direct or indirect effects, risks or hazards to herself or her unborn or newborn infant which may result from the use of a drug or procedure prescribed for or administered to her during pregnancy, labor, birth or lactation.

2. *The Pregnant Patient has the right,* prior to the proposed therapy, to be informed, not only of the benefits, risks and hazards of the proposed therapy but also of known alternative therapy, such as available childbirth education classes which could help to prepare the Pregnant Patient physically and mentally to cope with the discomfort or stress of pregnancy and the experience of childbirth, thereby reducing or eliminating her need for drugs and obstetric intervention. She should be offered such information early in her pregnancy in order that she may make a reasoned decision.

3. *The Pregnant Patient has the right,* prior to the administration of any drug, to be informed by the health professional who is prescribing or administering the drug to her that any drug which she receives during pregnancy, labor and birth, no matter how or when the drug is taken or administered, may adversely affect her unborn baby, directly or indirectly, and that there is no drug or chemical which has been proven safe for the unborn child.

4. *The Pregnant Patient has the right,* if Cesarean birth is anticipated, to be informed prior to the administration of any drug, and preferably prior to her hospitalization, that minimizing her and, in turn, her baby's intake of nonessential pre-operative medicine will benefit her baby.

5. *The Pregnant Patient has the right,* prior to the administration of a drug or procedure, to be informed of the areas of uncer-

tainty if there is NO properly controlled follow-up research which has established the safety of the drug or procedure with regard to its direct and/or indirect effects on the physiological, mental and neurological development of the child exposed, via the mother, to the drug or procedure during pregnancy, labor, birth or lactation — (this would apply to virtually all drugs and the majority of obstetric procedures).

6. *The Pregnant Patient has the right,* prior to the administration of any drug, to be informed of the brand name and generic name of the drug in order that she may advise the health professional of any past adverse reaction to the drug.

7. *The Pregnant Patient has the right* to determine for herself, without pressure from her attendant, whether she will accept the risks inherent in the proposed therapy or refuse a drug or procedure.

8. *The Pregnant Patient has the right* to know the name and qualifications of the individual administering a medication or procedure to her during labor or birth.

9. *The Pregnant Patient has the right* to be informed, prior to the administration of any procedure, whether that procedure is being administered to her for her or her baby's benefit (medically indicated) or as an elective procedure (for convenience, teaching purposes or research).

10. *The Pregnant Patient has the right* to be accompanied during the stress of labor and birth by someone she cares for, and to whom she looks for emotional comfort and encouragement.

11. *The Pregnant Patient has the right,* after appropriate medical consultation, to choose a position for labor and for birth which is least stressful to her baby and to herself.

12. *The Obstetric Patient has the right* to have her baby cared for at her bedside if her baby is normal, and to feed her baby according to her baby's needs rather than according to the hospital regimen.

13. *The Obstetric Patient has the right* to be informed in writing of the name of the person who actually delivered her baby and the professional qualifications of that person. This information should also be on the birth certificate.

14. *The Obstetric Patient has the right* to be informed if there is any known or indicated aspect of her or her baby's care or con-

dition which may cause her or her baby later difficulty or problems.

15. *The Obstetric Patient has the right* to have her and her baby's hospital medical records complete, accurate and legible and to have their records, including Nurses' Notes, retained by the hospital until the child reaches at least the age of majority, or, alternatively, to have the records offered to her before they are destroyed.

16. *The Obstetric Patient*, both during and after her hospital stay, has the right to have access to her complete hospital medical records, including Nurses' Notes, and to receive a copy upon payment of a reasonable fee and without incurring the expense of retaining an attorney.

It is the obstetric patient and her baby, not the health professional, who must sustain any trauma or injury resulting from the use of a drug or obstetric procedure. The observation of the rights listed above will not only permit the obstetric patient to participate in the decisions involving her and her baby's health care, but will help to protect the health professional and the hospital against litigation arising from resentment or misunderstanding on the part of the mother.

The Pregnant Patient's Responsibilities

In addition to understanding her rights the Pregnant Patient should also understand that she too has certain responsibilities. The Pregnant Patient's responsibilities include the following:

1. The Pregnant Patient is responsible for learning about the physical and psychological process of labor, birth and postpartum recovery. The better informed expectant parents are the better they will be able to participate in decisions concerning the planning of their care.

2. The Pregnant Patient is responsible for learning what comprises good prenatal and intranatal care and for making an effort to obtain the best care possible.

3. Expectant parents are responsible for knowing about those hospital policies and regulations which will affect their birth and postpartum experience.

4. The Pregnant Patient is responsible for arranging for a companion or support person (husband, mother, sister, friend, etc.) who will share in her plans for birth and who will accompany her during her labor and birth experience.

5. The Pregnant Patient is responsible for making her preferences known clearly to the health professionals involved in her case in a courteous and cooperative manner and for making mutually agreed-upon arrangements regarding maternity care alternatives with her physician and hospital in advance of labor.

6. Expectant parents are responsible for listening to their chosen physician or midwife with an open mind, just as they expect him or her to listen openly to them.

7. Once they have agreed to a course of health care, expectant parents are responsible, to the best of their ability, for seeing that the program is carried out in consultation with others with whom they have made the agreement.

8. The Pregnant Patient is responsible for obtaining information in advance regarding the approximate cost of her obstetric and hospital care.

9. The Pregnant Patient who intends to change her physician or hospital is responsible for notifying all concerned, well in advance of the birth if possible, and for informing both of her reasons for changing.

10. In all their interactions with medical and nursing personnel, the expectant parents should behave towards those caring for them with the same respect and consideration they themselves would like.

11. During the mother's hospital stay the mother is responsible for learning about her and her baby's continuing care after discharge from the hospital.

12. After birth, the parents should put into writing constructive comments and feelings of satisfaction and/or dissatisfaction with the care (nursing, medical and personal) they received. Good service to families in the future will be facilitated by those parents who take the time and responsibility to write letters expressing their feelings about the maternity care they received.

All the previous statements assume a normal birth and postpartum experience. Expectant parents should realize that, if complications develop in their cases, there will be an increased need to trust the expertise of the physician and hospital staff they have chosen. However, if problems occur, the childbearing woman still retains her responsibility for making informed decisions about her care or treatment and that of her baby. If she is incapable of assuming that responsibility because of her physical condition, her previously authorized companion or support person should assume responsibility for making informed decisions on her behalf.

Birth Plan

Below is a checklist of choices in childbirth. Expectant parents should discuss each option with their midwife or doctor, and place a copy of the plan in the mother's medical record.

Which of these are routines and which are options in your hospital or birth center? Most parents choose some options from each list.

MEDICAL PATHWAY	PHYSIOLOGIC PATHWAY
LABOR	**LABOR**
• Mother in wheelchair upon arrival at hospital.	• Mother walks to labor and delivery.
• Shave, minishave, or clipping of long hairs on perineum.	• No shave or clipping of hair.
• Enema.	• Bowels emptied spontaneously, or enema self-administered at home.
• Partner is asked to leave during prep and exams.	• Partner present throughout labor & delivery.
• Limit to one support person during labor and birth.	• Presence of other friends, relatives, and siblings.
• Confinement to bed and/or one position.	• Freedom to walk and change positions as desired.
• Induction of labor. Methods: Stripping membranes, amniotomy, oxytocin.	• Spontaneous labor. Alternatives: Making love, breast stimulation.
• IV fluids for hydration and energy.	• Drinking fluid or eating as desired.
• Frequent vaginal exams.	• Vaginal exams when requested by mother or for medical reasons.
• Electronic fetal heart monitor.	• Listening to fetal heart with fetal stethoscope.
• Pain relief through medication: analgesics or anesthetics.	• Relaxation, emotional support, massage, breathing.
BIRTH	**BIRTH**
• Lithotomy position or semisitting in labor bed for pushing.	• Choice of position and freedom to move.
• Prolonged breath-holding and bearing down for expulsion.	• Mother follows her urge to push, vocalizing if she wishes.
• Limit of two hours on 2nd stage — then forceps or caesarean birth.	• Allow for longer 2nd stage and position variations to help progress.
• Delivery table for birth.	• Birth in labor bed, birth chair, or beanbag.
• Lithotomy position with stirrups for birth.	• Side-lying, all fours, squatting, standing with leg up, semireclining with back support, no stirrups.
• Mother not allowed to touch sterile field.	• Mother allowed to touch baby's head as it crowns.
• Catheterization in 2nd stage.	• No catheterization and frequent voiding in first stage.
• Episiotomy.	• No episiotomy: massage, warm compresses, slower delivery, coaching to pant out baby, support to perineum. Late episiotomy with no anesthesia.
• Forceps or vacuum extraction.	• Spontaneous delivery.

The complete pamphlet "Planning Your Baby's Birth" is available in single copies (50 cents) or bulk orders ($20 per 100, includes postage and handling) from the pennypress, 1100 23rd Ave. East, Seattle, WA 98112.

AFTERBIRTH	AFTERBIRTH
• Intubation/suctioning.	• Waiting to see if baby can handle own mucus.
• Immediate care of baby done out of sight of mother: e.g., identification, Apgar, heat lamp, replace hemostat with cord clamp.	• Care done on mother's abdomen. Baby skin to skin with mother with heat lamp or blanket over them. Delay in nonessential routines.
• Limit of 15–20 minutes on 3rd stage followed by manual extraction of the placenta.	• Allow for longer time for placenta. Allow mother to move around, nurse baby. Let cord drain.
• Pitocin drip or injection for contraction of uterus after placenta is born.	• Evaluation of uterus before using uterine stimulant routinely. Breastfeeding.

BABY	BABY
• Baby to isolette or nursery for 4–24 hours. Mother to recovery room for observation.	• Baby held by mother or father on delivery table and/or in recovery.
• Eye drops — silver nitrate applied shortly after birth.	• Omit eye drops or delay administration up to 2 hours. Use of other agent as alternative.
• Baby's first feeding — glucose water by nurse.	• Colostrum by mother who plans to breastfeed or plain water given by mother.
• Baby in nursery except for scheduled 4-hour feedings.	• Demand feeding, baby to mother when crying. Twenty-four-hour rooming-in.
• Circumcision.	• No circumcision, or parents present to comfort baby after operation.
• Home in 3 or more days after delivery.	• Early discharge from hospital.

THE UNEXPECTED

COMMON MEDICAL PROCEDURES	POSSIBLE OPTIONS
CAESAREAN BIRTH	CAESAREAN BIRTH
• Scheduled surgery.	• Surgery after labor begins.
• Mother without her support person in surgery.	• Father present to support mother.
• General anesthesia.	• Spinal or epidural.
• Screen to prevent viewing surgery.	• Screen lowered at time of birth or baby held up for mother and father to see.
• Mother not allowed to wear contacts or glasses.	• Mother to wear contacts or glasses.
• Baby sent to intensive care nursery.	• Father to hold baby and mother to see baby, if baby is not in distress. Mother allowed to breastfeed in recovery if her and her baby's condition permit.

PREMATURE/SICK INFANT	PREMATURE/SICK INFANT
• Baby cared for by professionals.	• Parents involved in care of baby, diapering, touching, talking to baby in incubator, feeding baby.
• Baby rushed to intensive care.	• Mother allowed to hold and see baby, if not distressed.
• Baby sent to another hospital or another part of hospital.	• Baby close to mother; in same part of hospital.
• Baby transported to hospital with intensive care unit.	• Father goes with the transport team, mother goes if she is able.
• Limited visits to baby from mother only.	• Father and/or extended family allowed to see baby.
• IV and bottle feeding.	• Mother allowed to express her colostrum for the baby and encouraged and helped to get started at breastfeeding.

Authorities Quoted

Swami Ajaya, formerly known as Alan Weinstock, is a clinical psychologist and author of *Yoga Psychology*.

Grantly Dick-Read, M.D., was an English obstetrician and the "father of natural childbirth." His classic *Childbirth Without Fear,* published in 1933, was the first book on birth written for mothers.

Ken Dychtwald is a psychologist, founding president of the Association for Humanistic Gerontology, and author of *Bodymind*.

Moshe Feldenkrais is an Israeli physicist and author who developed the Feldenkrais method of body-mind exercises.

Marilyn Ferguson is the author of *The Aquarian Conspiracy* and the publisher of *Brain/Mind Bulletin*.

Chloe Fisher is a midwife in Oxford, England.

Erich Fromm is a psychoanalyst and the author of many books, including *Escape from Freedom, Man for Himself,* and *The Art of Loving*.

Ina May Gaskin is the author of *Spiritual Midwifery* and chief midwife at The Farm, a self-sufficient community in Tennessee.

Doris Haire is the president of the American Foundation for Maternal and Child Health and author of many articles on breastfeeding, drugs, and obstetrics, including *The Cultural Warping of Childbirth*.

Oliver Wendell Holmes, M.D., a nineteenth-century physician and author of essays and poems, is best known for his "Breakfast-Table" papers.

Aldous Huxley was a member of the illustrious British family of scientists and writers. His books include *Brave New World, The Doors of Perception,* and *Island.*

Ivan Illich is an Austrian writer of powerful social criticism. His books include *DeSchooling Society, Tools for Conviviality,* and *Medical Nemesis.*

B. K. S. Iyengar, an Indian yoga practitioner of great repute, is the author of *Light on Yoga.* Many of his axioms have been compiled in *Sparks of Divinity* by Noelle Perez-Christaens.

Joel Kramer, an accomplished American yogi, is the author of *The Passionate Mind.*

R. D. Laing, Scottish psychiatrist, is the author of many books, including *The Facts of Life* and *The Divided Self.* He is also the narrator of a powerful film critique of modern obstetrics, *Birth with R. D. Laing.*

Lao Tzu was a Chinese poet and philosopher born in 604 B.C. His famous reflections are compiled in *The Way of Life.*

Judith Lasater is a physical therapist and a founder of *Yoga Journal* and the Institute of Yoga Teacher Education in San Francisco.

Frederick Leboyer, M.D., is the French obstetrician who first drew international attention to the insensitive handling of the newborn with his book and film *Birth Without Violence.*

Alexander Lowen, M.D., is a psychiatrist who popularized the therapy of Bioenergetics, based on Wilhelm Reich's work.

Abraham Maslow is a psychologist and author of many books, including *Toward a Psychology of Being.*

Ashley Montagu is an anthropologist and prolific writer whose books include *Touching* and *Life Before Birth.*

Frederick (Fritz) Perls, a psychotherapist, brought the theory of Gestalt psychology from Germany to the U.S. He is the author of *Gestalt Therapy Verbatim* and *Gestalt Therapy: Excitement and Growth in the Human Personality.*

Eva Reich, M.D., is an international lecturer on birth, infant massage, and Bioenergetics. She is the daughter of Wilhelm Reich.

Wilhelm Reich was an Austrian psychiatrist who developed the theory of cosmic orgone energy and first described how emotional tensions cause bodily "armoring." His writings include *The Function of the Orgasm* and *The Murder of Christ.*

Paul Reps, an American who has lived in the East, is the author of several books of poems and prose, including *Zen Flesh, Zen Bones.*

Carl Rogers, a psychologist, is the author of many books and articles on psychotherapy, including *On Becoming a Person.*

Leni Schwartz is an environmental psychologist and author of *The World of the Unborn.*

Shu Ching was a sixth-century Chinese philosopher.

Frans Veldman is the founder and director of the Society for the Research and Development of Haptonomy (the science of touch) in France.

Alan Watts was a theologian and philosopher known for introducing the West to Zen Buddhism and Indian and Chinese philosophy. He died in 1973. His books include *Nature, Man and Woman* and *The Wisdom of Insecurity.*

Max Weber, a German sociologist and political economist, wrote many books, including *The Protestant Ethic and The Spirit of Capitalism.*

Kerr L. White is director of the Rockefeller Foundation of Health Sciences.

Ludwig Wittgenstein was an Austrian engineer and philosopher most noted for his *Tractatus-Logico Philosophicus.*

Diony Young is a consultant for the International Childbirth Education Association and author of several books and articles, including *Bonding* and *Unnecessary Cesareans — Ways to Prevent Them.*

Bibliography

Books

Alexander, F. Matthias. *The Resurrection of the Body.* New York: Dell, 1974.

Basmajian, J. D. *Muscles Alive: Their Functions as Revealed by Electromyography.* 4th ed. Baltimore: Williams and Wilkins, 1980.

Betherat, Therese, and Carol Bernstein. *The Body Has Its Reasons: Anti-Exercises and Self-Awareness.* New York: Avon, 1978.

Bradley, Robert, M.D. *Husband-Coached Childbirth.* New York: Harper and Row, 1974.

Bronowski, Jacob. *The Ascent of Man.* Boston: Little, Brown, 1974.

Brown, Barbara B. *New Mind, New Body.* New York: Bantam, 1974.

Buxton, R. St. J. *Maternal Respiration in Labour: An Initial Comparative Study of the Effects of Various Ante-Natal Training Programs.* London: Obstetric Association of Chartered Physiotherapists, 14 Bedford Row, London WC1, 1969.

Crookall, Robert. *Psychic Breathing.* Wellingsborough, Northamptonshire, U.K.: Aquarian Press, 1979.

Dick-Read, Grantly. *Childbirth Without Fear.* Rev. ed. New York: Harper and Row, 1979.

Dychtwald, Ken. *Bodymind.* New York: Random House, 1977.

Farson, Richard. *Birthrights.* New York: Macmillan, 1974.

Feitis, Rosemary, ed. *Ida Rolf Talks: About Rolfing and Physical Reality.* New York: Harper and Row, 1978.

Feldenkrais, Moshe. *Body and Mature Behavior*. New York: International Universities Press, Inc., 1949.

———. *Awareness Through Movement*. New York: Harper and Row, 1972.

———. *The Case of Nora*. New York: Harper and Row, 1977.

———. *The Elusive Obvious*. Cupertino, Calif.: Meta Publications, 1981.

Fraiberg, Selma. *Every Child's Birth Right: In Defense of Mothering*. New York: Bantam, 1977.

Funderburk, James, Ph.D. *Science Studies Yoga: A Review of Physiological Data*. Honesdale, Penn.: Himalayan Institute of Yoga Science and Philosophy, 1977.

Gaskin, Ina May. *Spiritual Midwifery*. Summertown, Tenn.: Book Publishing Company, 1982.

Grof, Stanislav. *Realms of the Human Unconscious: Observations from LSD Research*. New York: Dutton, 1976.

Haire, Doris. *The Cultural Warping of Childbirth*. ICEA Publication, P.O. Box 20048, Minneapolis, MN 55420.

Henderson, Joe. *Run Gently, Run Long*. Mountain View, Calif.: World Publications, 1975.

Illich, Ivan. *Medical Nemesis*. New York: Bantam, 1977.

Jackson, Ian. *Yoga and the Athlete*. Mountain View, Calif.: World Publications, 1975.

Karmel, Marjorie. *Thank You, Dr. Lamaze*. New York: Lippincott, 1959.

Kitzinger, Sheila, and John Davis, eds. *Birth at Home*. Oxford, UK: Oxford University Press, 1978.

Kramer, Joel. *The Passionate Mind: A Manual for Living Creatively with One's Self*. Millbrae, Calif.: Celestial Arts, 1974.

Kuhn, T. S. *The Structure of Scientific Revolutions*. Chicago: University of Chicago Press, 1962.

Laing, R. D. *The Facts of Life*. New York: Pantheon, 1976.

Lamaze, Fernand. *Painless Childbirth: The Lamaze Method*. New York: Pocket, 1972.

Lowen, Alexander. *Bioenergetics*. New York: Penguin, 1975.

———. *The Betrayal of the Body*. New York: Macmillan, 1969.

———. *Depression and the Body*. New York: Penguin, 1977.

Lumley, Judith, and Jill Astbury. *Birth Rites, Birth Rights.* Melbourne, Australia: Sphere, 1980.

Maltz, Maxwell, M.D. *Psycho-Cybernetics.* New York: Pocket, 1960.

Maslow, Abraham. *Toward a Psychology of Being.* 2nd ed. Van Nostrand Reinhold, 1968.

———. *The Farther Reaches of Human Nature.* New York: Penguin, 1976.

McCall, Robert. *Infants.* New York: Random House, 1980.

Montagu, Ashley. *Life Before Birth.* New York: Signet, 1977.

Ornstein, Robert. *The Psychology of Consciousness.* New York: Harcourt Brace Jovanovich, 1972.

Orr, Leonard, and Sondra Ray. *Rebirthing in the New Age.* Millbrae, Calif.: Celestial Arts, 1977.

Ouspensky, P. D. *A New Model of the Universe.* New York: Random House, 1971.

Passmore, John. *A Hundred Years of Philosophy.* Baltimore, Md.: Penguin, 1966.

Perez-Christaens, Noelle. *Sparks of Divinity.* Paris: Institute de Yoga B. K. S. Iyengar, 72, Avenue alta Bourdonnais, 1976.

Perls, Frederick, Ralph Hefferline, and Paul Goodman. *Gestalt Therapy: Excitement and Growth in the Human Personality.* New York: Bantam Books, 1977.

Swami Rama, Rudolph Ballentine, and Alan Hymes. *The Science of Breath: A Practical Guide.* Honesdale, Penn.: Himalayan Institute of Yoga Science and Philosophy, 1979.

Swami Rama, Rudolph Ballentine, and Swami Ajaya. *Yoga and Psychotherapy — The Evolution of Consciousness.* Honesdale, Penn.: Himalayan Institute of Yoga Science and Philosophy, 1976.

Reich, Wilhelm. *The Function of the Orgasm.* trans. Vincent R. Carfagno. New York: Simon and Schuster, 1973.

Reps, Paul. *Juicing.* Garden City, N.Y.: Doubleday, 1978.

Revolutionary Health Care Committee of Hunan Province. *A Barefoot Doctor's Manual: A Guide to Traditional Chinese and Modern Medicine.* Mayne Isle and Seattle: Cloudburst Press, 1977.

Rogers, Carl. *On Becoming a Person.* Boston: Houghton Mifflin, 1961.

Sagan, Carl. *Cosmos*. New York: Random House, 1980.

Shoemaker, Sydney. *Self-Knowledge and Self-Identity*. Ithaca, N.Y.: Cornell University Press, 1963.

Simonton, O. Carl, M.D., Stephanie Matthews-Simonton, and James L. Creighton. *Getting Well Again*. New York: Bantam, 1978.

Vellay, Pierre. *Childbirth Without Pain*. London: Allen and Unwin, 1959.

Watts, Alan. *The Wisdom of Insecurity*. New York: Random House, 1951.

———. *Psychotherapy — East and West*. New York: Vintage, 1961.

———. *Nature, Man and Woman*. New York: Random House, 1970.

———. *The Book: On the Taboo Against Knowing Who You Are*. New York: Random House, 1972.

Weil, Andrew T. *The Marriage of the Sun and Moon: A Quest for Unity in Consciousness*. Boston: Houghton Mifflin, 1981.

Young, Diony. *Bonding: How Parents Become Attached to Their Child*. ICEA, Box 20048, Minneapolis, MN 55420, 1978.

———. *Unnecessary Cesareans — Ways to Prevent Them*. ICEA, Box 20048, Minneapolis, MN 55420, 1980.

———. *Changing Childbirth*. Rochester, N.Y.: Childbirth Graphics, 1982.

Articles

Beynon, Constance. "The Normal Second Stage of Labor." *Journal of Obstetrics and Gynaecology of the British Empire* 64 (December 1957): 815–20.

Cohen, H. D., D. Goodenough, H. A. Witkin, P. Oltman, H. Gould, and E. Shulman. "The Effects of Stress on Components of the Respiratory Cycle." *Psychophysiology* 12:4 (1975): 377–380.

Dunn, P. "Obstetric Delivery Today: For Better or For Worse?" *Lancet* 1:7963 (April 1976).

Ehrstrom, Chr. "Forlossingstolar." Reprint from *Recip Reflex* 13, 72 (1973), cited in Kirchoff, H. "The Woman's Posture During

Childbirth." *Organorama* 14:1. (Organanon, Oss, The Netherlands.)

Ferguson, J. K. W. "A Study of the Motility of the Intact Uterus at Term." *Surgery, Gynecology and Obstetrics* 73 (1941): 359–366.

Fisher, Chloe. "The Management of Labour: A Midwife's View." In *Episiotomy: Physical and Emotional Aspects,* ed. Sheila Kitzinger. London: National Childbirth Trust, 9 Queensborough Terrace, London, W.2, 1981.

Flynn, A. M., J. Kelly, F. Hollins, P. F. Lynch. "Ambulation in Labour." *British Medical Journal* 2 (August 26, 1978): 591–93.

Harris, C., E. Katkin, J. Lick, T. Habberfield. "Paced Respiration as a Technique for the Modification of Autonomic Response to Stress." *Psychophysiology* 13:5 (September 1976).

Holmes, D. S., K. D. McCaul, S. Solomon. "Control of Respiration as a Means of Controlling Responses to Threat." *Journal of Personality and Social Psychology* 36:2 (1978): 198–204.

Humphrey, M. D., A. Chang, E. C. Wood, S. Morgan, D. Hounslow. "A Decrease in Fetal pH During the Second Stage of Labour When Conducted in the Dorsal Position." *Journal of Obstetrics and Gynaecology of the British Commonwealth* 81:600 (1974).

Morgan, W. "The Mind of the Marathoners." *Psychology Today,* April 1978.

Sosa, Roberto, John Kennell, Marshall Klaus, Steven Robertson, and Juan Urrutia. "The Effect of a Supportive Companion on Perinatal Problems, Length of Labor and Maternal-Infant Attachment." *New England Journal of Medicine* 303:11 (September 11, 1980): 597–600.

Index